The NoPause Solution Handbook

A Physician's Integrative Guide Through Perimenopause and Menopause

Ivanah Thomas, MD

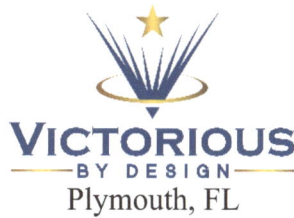

VICTORIOUS
—BY DESIGN—
Plymouth, FL

MEDICAL DISCLAIMER

The information in this book is provided for educational, informational, and inspirational purposes only. It is not intended to replace a one-on-one relationship with a qualified healthcare professional or to serve as individualized medical, diagnostic, or treatment advice.

While Dr. Thomas is a physician, the guidance in this book is general in nature and may not be appropriate for every reader's unique health situation. Always consult your physician or another qualified healthcare provider regarding any questions you have about your symptoms, medical conditions, treatments, supplements, or changes to your health, diet, or lifestyle.

Never ignore or delay seeking professional medical advice because of something you have read in this book. If you are experiencing a medical emergency, call your healthcare provider or emergency services immediately.

The author and publisher disclaim any liability for any loss, injury, or adverse outcome resulting directly or indirectly from the use or application of the information presented in this publication.

Published by Victorious By Design
Plymouth, Florida.

ISBN-13: 978-1-7332347-5-7
ISBN-10: 1-7332347-5-6

For more information about this book, please contact:

Victorious By Design
P.O. Box 638
Plymouth, FL 32768
www.victoriousbydesign.com

Cover design by Keron Williams

Printed in the United States of America

DEDICATION

To every woman who has ever felt unseen, unheard, or misunderstood during her perimenopausal or menopausal journey, this book is for you. May you discover strength, clarity, and the confidence to thrive in every season of your life.

TABLE OF CONTENTS

AUTHOR'S NOTE

As you begin this book, I want you to know one thing above all else: you are not imagining what you are feeling, and you are not alone. The changes you may be experiencing, whether physical, emotional, or cognitive, can feel confusing and overwhelming. But they are real, they are valid, and they deserve to be understood with compassion and clarity.

This handbook was written with you in mind. It is designed to be a companion, a resource you can return to again and again, whether you are just starting to notice changes or are well into your transition. My hope is that as you read, you will feel seen, supported, and empowered to take an active role in your health.

You will find practical strategies, evidence-based guidance, and integrative approaches that I have used both personally and professionally to help women navigate this season with confidence. You will also find encouragement, because knowledge without hope can feel heavy, but knowledge with hope can transform your life.

Perimenopause and menopause are not signs of decline. They are an invitation to reset, to reevaluate, to nourish yourself in ways you may have never prioritized before. This season is not something to endure in silence. It is something you can move through with strength, understanding, and even renewed purpose.

Thank you for trusting me to walk alongside you. May these pages bring you clarity, comfort, and the reassurance that you were never meant to navigate this alone.

Ivanah Thomas, MD

INTRODUCTION
The Transition No One Prepared You For

The Night Everything Changed

It was 3:47 AM, when forty-six-year-old Sarah woke up drenched in sweat, her heart pounding, her nightgown soaked through. For a moment, she wondered if she was getting sick; had she caught a virus? Was something seriously wrong? Then she remembered: this was the third night this week.

The next morning, exhausted from yet another disrupted night, she forgot her colleague's name mid-sentence during a presentation. The woman she had worked with for five years. Sarah stumbled through the rest of the meeting, her face appeared flushed with embarrassment or was that another hot flash? She could not tell anymore. Later that afternoon, her husband made an innocuous comment about dinner plans, and Sarah found herself inexplicably angry, snapping at him with an intensity that surprised them both. By evening, the anger had dissolved into tears. What was happening to her?

If you have picked up this book, Sarah's story probably sounds familiar. Maybe you are waking up drenched in sweat. Maybe you are forgetting words, feeling like you are thinking through cotton, or wondering if you are developing early-onset dementia. Maybe your periods have become unpredictable; flooding one month, absent the next. Maybe you are experiencing mood swings that make you feel like you are losing your mind, or anxiety that seems to come from nowhere and everywhere at once. Maybe you feel like your body has been hijacked by some force you do not understand, and you are desperately seeking answers, while silently hoping that you will feel like yourself again.

Welcome. You have come to the right place.

The Moment That Changed Everything For Me

I will never forget the day I nearly fainted in the operating room. I was almost at the end of a procedure; my hands steady, my focus sharp, doing what I had been trained to do, when suddenly, a wave of heat erupted from my mid chest and converged on my face. My surgical mask felt suffocating. Sweat pooled under my gown. My vision blurred at the edges, and for a terrifying moment, I thought I might collapse right there over my patient. I quickly said to my colleague, "Doc, I feel like I'm going to pass out." With a look of grave concern she stated, "what?" The anesthesiologist instinctively stepped behind me and caught me before I fell. I was placed on a stretcher and carried out to a private room where my colleagues tended to me with utmost care and compassion. I was shaken to my core and embarrassed as waves of emotions engulfed me.

This was not the first time that I experienced intense hot flashes, but it certainly was the worst one. The hot flashes had been happening for months, sudden, overwhelming, and impossible to predict. They struck during surgeries, during patient consultations, during meetings. They woke me up at night, my sheets soaked through, my heart pounding. I was exhausted, irritable, and struggling to concentrate.

I was at the peak of my career, and I felt like I was falling apart. Looking back, I realize how little attention we had given to menopause in my medical training. Maybe a lecture or two. A brief mention in an OB-GYN rotation. Nothing that prepared me to recognize it in myself, let alone help my patients navigate it effectively.

That moment in the operating room changed everything. It did not just change how I felt about my symptoms; it changed the entire trajectory of my medical career. I realized I could not continue this way, my patients deserved better, and so did I. I needed to understand what was happening to my body, why it was happening, and what I could do about it.

I dove deep into research on perimenopause and menopause, studying hormones, integrative medicine, and evidence-based natural approaches. I explored not just what conventional medicine offered, but what emerging science revealed about nutrition, supplements, lifestyle interventions, and holistic support. The more I learned, the more I understood how profoundly these hormonal changes affect every system in our bodies, and how inadequately most women are supported through this transition.

This research journey led me to develop two nutraceutical products that have transformed my own life: NoPause Hot Flashes Support and NoPause Mood Support, for brain fog, mood swings, irritability, night sweats, and insomnia. These formulations gave me my zest for life back, that vitality and clarity I thought I had lost forever. Even more rewarding, these products have transformed the lives of countless women on their perimenopause and menopause journey, from the USA and Canada to the UK, the Caribbean, and as far as South Africa.

The Conversation We Should Have Had Years Ago

Here is what is stunning: all women will go through menopause, yet most women enter perimenopause, the transition leading up to menopause, with almost no understanding of what is happening to them. We are given the "facts of life" talk as teenagers about menstruation and reproduction. We receive countless messages about pregnancy, childbirth, and motherhood. But about this transition, this significant life passage that can span a decade and affect every aspect of our physical, mental, and emotional health? Silence.

This silence is not benign, it is costly, both physically and economically. At any given time, approximately twenty five percent of the workforce is experiencing perimenopause or menopause symptoms. This impacts their productivity and well-being. Approximately fifty percent have symptoms that disrupts their work, leading to reduced performance, and increased health costs. Globally, worker productivity losses due to menopausal symptoms are estimated at $150 billion annually, with related healthcare costs exceeding $600 billion. In the United States alone, the economy loses $26.6 billion each year from failing to accommodate menopause, with an additional $1.8 billion in lost productivity from missed work days.

These numbers represent real women struggling in silence. Women who spend an average of $2,100 annually on healthcare costs related to their transition. Women who miss up to fourteen days of work per year due to symptoms. Women who earn ten percent less four years after seeking medical help for menopausal symptoms.

The personal toll is even more devastating. This silence leaves women confused, frightened, and suffering unnecessarily. It causes women to attribute menopausal symptoms to other causes, stress, aging, depression, or worse, to think they are "going crazy." It keeps women from seeking help because they do not realize their symptoms are related to hormonal changes. And it prevents women from accessing treatments and strategies that could dramatically improve their quality of life during this transition.

Perhaps most troubling: ninety-nine percent of women going through menopause receive no workplace support or benefits related to their symptoms. They are expected to simply power through one of the most significant biological transitions of their lives without acknowledgment, accommodation, or assistance.

The silence around menopause reflects a broader cultural discomfort with aging women. In a society that equates women's value with youth, fertility, and conventional attractiveness, menopause, which signals the end of reproductive years, becomes something to hide, deny, or simply not discuss. Women become complicit in this silence, often suffering alone rather than talking openly about their experiences.

But the silence is breaking. Women are increasingly refusing to accept that this significant life transition should be shrouded in secrecy and shame. We are talking to each other, sharing our experiences, demanding better from healthcare providers, and insisting on information, support, and effective treatment. We are recognizing that this is not just a personal health issue, it is an economic issue, a workplace issue, and a social justice issue. This book is part of that conversation.

Why I Wrote This Book

I wrote this book because of my own personal journey and the fulfillment I have found by utilizing some of these strategies in this book. I have seen too many women suffer unnecessarily through perimenopause and menopause. I have worked with countless women who spent months or years struggling with symptoms before anyone, including themselves, connected those symptoms to hormonal changes.

I have also seen the transformation that occurs when women receive accurate information, appropriate support, and effective treatment. I have watched women reclaim their sleep, their cognitive function, their emotional stability, and their sense of self. I have seen women implement lifestyle changes that not only ease their menopausal transition but also lay the foundation for decades of vibrant health. I have witnessed women emerge from this transition stronger, clearer, and more authentically themselves than they have ever been.

Every woman deserves this kind of support. Every woman deserves to navigate this transition with knowledge, appropriate care, and the understanding that feeling better is possible. This book aims to provide that support, in an accessible, evidence-based way.

This book is also for the partners, family members, and friends of women going through this transition, and want to understand and support the women they love.

What You Will Learn Next

In the chapters that follow, you will learn how hormones shift, why symptoms occur, and the integrative strategies that can restore balance, vitality, and emotional wellbeing. You will discover tools you can begin using right away, insights that help you understand your body more deeply, and evidence-based approaches to guide you toward feeling like yourself again.

PART I

UNDERSTANDING WHAT'S HAPPENING

CHAPTER 1

Perimenopause vs. Menopause - What's the Difference?

The confusion is undeniable. Most of us grew up hearing about "menopause" as this singular event that happens to women in their 50s. Hot flashes. No more periods. Done.

The reality is far more complex, and understanding the difference between perimenopause and menopause is crucial for getting the right treatment at the right time.

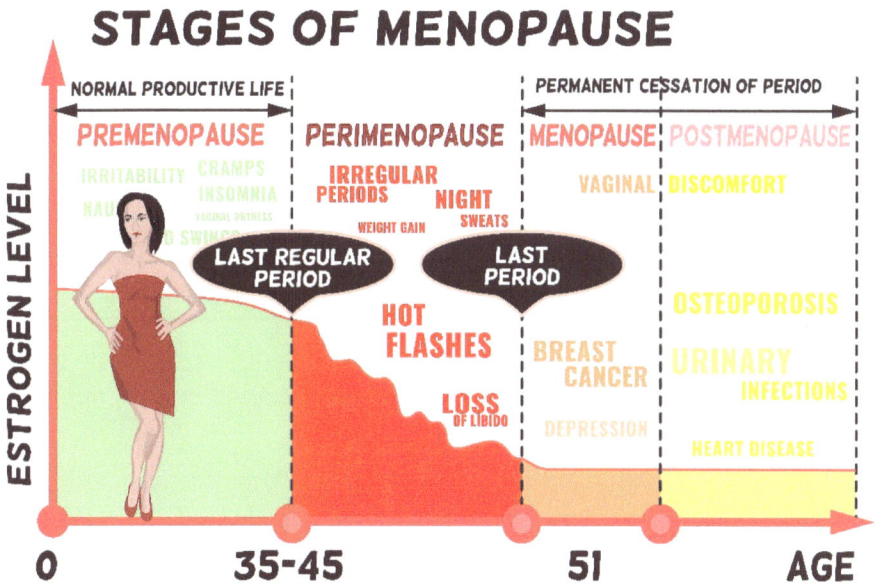

STAGES OF MENOPAUSE

The Three Stages: A Journey, Not a Destination

Think of your reproductive life as having distinct phases. You moved through puberty into your reproductive years. Now you are transitioning out of them. Just as puberty was not a single day but a multi-year process, so is the transition into menopause.

There are three stages you need to understand:

1. PERIMENOPAUSE: The Transition Years

What it is: Perimenopause means "around menopause." It is the transitional period when your ovaries gradually produce less estrogen and progesterone. Your body is shifting from reproductive to post-reproductive, but it is not a smooth, linear decline. Instead, hormones fluctuate wildly, sometimes high, often low, rarely stable.

When it starts: Most women enter perimenopause in their 40s, but it can begin as early as your mid-30s. The average age is 45, but "average" means very little when every woman's timeline is unique.

How long it lasts: Typically, 4-8 years, but it can be as short as a few months or as long as 10+ years. I know that is a frustratingly wide range. Your genetics, lifestyle, stress levels, and overall health all play a role.

What is happening: Your ovaries are still functioning, but inconsistently. Some months you ovulate normally. Other months you do not. Estrogen levels swing dramatically, sometimes higher than ever, sometimes crashing. Progesterone, which you only produce after ovulation, becomes increasingly deficient.

Your periods: This is where it gets confusing. Your menstrual cycle during perimenopause can do almost anything:

- Shorter cycles (21-24 days instead of 28)
- Longer cycles (35-60+ days)
- Heavier bleeding
- Lighter bleeding
- Skipped periods followed by normal ones
- Irregular timing that makes planning anything difficult

The symptoms: This is when most women start feeling "off." Hot flashes, night sweats, palpitations, mood swings, anxiety, insomnia, brain fog, weight gain, joint pain, decreased libido, all the symptoms we associate with "menopause" typically starts in perimenopause. In fact, perimenopause is often when symptoms are worst because of the hormonal chaos.

Important: You can still get pregnant during perimenopause. Until you have gone 12 consecutive months without a period, ovulation is still possible. If you do not want to conceive, continue using birth control.

2. MENOPAUSE: The Single Day

What it is: Menopause is technically a single moment in time, the point at which you have gone 12 consecutive months without a menstrual period. It is diagnosed retrospectively. You can only confirm you have reached menopause after a full year without bleeding.

When it happens: The average age is 51, but anywhere from age 45-55 is considered normal. If menopause occurs before age 40, it is called premature menopause. Before age 45, it is early menopause. After 55, it is considered late onset menopause.

What is happening: Your ovaries have essentially stopped producing estrogen and progesterone. You are no longer ovulating. Your reproductive years have ended.

The symptoms: Interestingly, some women feel better once they reach menopause because their hormones, while low, are finally stable. The wild fluctuations of perimenopause have ended. However, other women continue experiencing symptoms, particularly hot flashes, vaginal dryness, and sleep disturbances, which brings us to....

3. POSTMENOPAUSE: The Rest of Your Life

What it is: Post-menopause is every year after menopause. Once you have reached that 12-month mark without a period, you are postmenopausal for the rest of your life.

What is happening: Your ovaries produce very little estrogen and progesterone. Your adrenal glands and fat tissue produce small amounts of hormones, but nothing like your reproductive years. This becomes your new normal.

The symptoms: Some women sail through post-menopause symptom-free. Others experience ongoing challenges. Hot flashes can persist for years (or even decades). Vaginal atrophy and painful intercourse often worsen without treatment. Bone density loss accelerates. Cardiovascular risk increases.

The good news: This is also when many women report feeling more confident, settled, and free. Without monthly hormonal fluctuations, moods often stabilize. Without worrying about periods or pregnancy, life becomes simpler. And with proper support, whether hormones, supplements, or lifestyle optimization, the physical symptoms are absolutely manageable.

Why the Terminology Matters

You might be thinking: "Does it really matter whether I call it perimenopause or menopause?"

Yes. It matters tremendously. Here is why:

Treatment timing is different. What works in perimenopause may differ from what is needed in post-menopause. For example, many perimenopausal women need progesterone more urgently than estrogen because they are still producing erratic estrogen but little to no progesterone. Postmenopausal women typically need both.

Testing interpretation is different. Hormone tests during perimenopause are notoriously unreliable because levels fluctuate daily. In post-menopause, they are more stable and useful for monitoring treatment.

Birth control matters in perimenopause but not post-menopause. Knowing which stage you are in affects family planning decisions.

How to Know Which Stage You're In

You are likely in PERIMENOPAUSE if:

- You are 35-55 years old with changing menstrual patterns
- Your cycles have become irregular (shorter, longer, skipped)
- You are experiencing symptoms like hot flashes, mood changes, or sleep problems
- You are still having some periods, even if unpredictable

You are in MENOPAUSE (the transition point) if:

- You have gone 12 consecutive months without any menstrual bleeding
- You are typically 45-55 years old (though age varies)

You are in POST-MENOPAUSE if:

- It has been more than 12 months since your last period
- You are no longer having any menstrual bleeding

Special situations:

If you have had a hysterectomy (uterus removed), determining your stage is trickier. If your ovaries were preserved, they will still go through perimenopause and menopause, you just will not have periods as a marker. Symptoms and age become your guide. If your ovaries were also removed, you immediately enter surgical menopause.

If you have had an endometrial ablation (a procedure that destroys the uterine lining), you may no longer menstruate even though your ovaries are still functioning. Again, symptoms and age help determine your stage. Below is a list of perimenopause and menopause symptoms. Most of these symptoms will be will be elaborated on in Chapter 3.

List of Possible Perimenopause and Menopause Symptoms:

Vasomotor Symptoms: • Hot flashes (sudden feelings of heat) • Night sweats • Hot flushes (reddening of skin with heat) • Cold flashes • Chills • Increased perspiration • Heat intolerance.

Sleep Disturbances: • Insomnia (difficulty falling asleep) • Difficulty staying asleep • Early morning awakening • Restless sleep • Vivid dreams or nightmares • Sleep apnea or worsening of existing sleep apnea • Disrupted sleep patterns • Excessive daytime sleepiness or fatigue.

Cognitive and Neurological Symptoms: • Brain fog (mental cloudiness) • Memory problems (short-term memory loss) • Difficulty concentrating • Mental confusion or disorientation • Difficulty with word retrieval • Decreased ability to multitask • Slower processing speed • Headaches (increased frequency or intensity) • Migraines (new onset or worsening) • Dizziness or lightheadedness • Vertigo • Burning tongue or mouth (burning mouth syndrome) • Changes in taste perception • Tinnitus (ringing in ears).

Mood and Emotional Symptoms: • Mood swings (rapid emotional changes) • Irritability • Anxiety (generalized or panic attacks) • Depression or depressive symptoms • Increased stress sensitivity • Emotional lability (crying easily) • Feelings of sadness or melancholy • Loss of motivation • Decreased self-esteem • Feelings of dread or apprehension • Social withdrawal • Increased anger or rage episodes.

Menstrual Changes: • Irregular periods (changes in cycle length) • Heavy menstrual bleeding (menorrhagia) • Light or skipped periods • Shorter or longer cycles • Spotting between periods • Longer or shorter duration of bleeding • Flooding (sudden heavy flow) • Blood clots during menstruation • Complete cessation of periods (amenorrhea).

Urogenital and Pelvic Symptoms: • Vaginal dryness • Vaginal atrophy (thinning of vaginal walls) • Vaginal irritation or burning • Painful intercourse (dyspareunia) • Decreased libido (low sex drive) • Loss of sexual desire • Difficulty achieving orgasm • Reduced sexual satisfaction • Urinary urgency • Urinary frequency (need to urinate often) • Urinary incontinence (stress or urge)   • Recurrent urinary tract infections (UTIs) • Painful urination (dysuria) • Bladder sensitivity • Pelvic floor weakness • Uterine prolapse or worsening prolapse.

Musculoskeletal Symptoms: • Joint pain (arthralgia) • Joint stiffness (especially morning stiffness) • Muscle aches and pains (myalgia) • Muscle tension • Back pain • Neck and shoulder pain • Frozen shoulder • Decreased flexibility • Osteoporosis or osteopenia (bone loss) • Increased risk of fractures • Tendonitis • Carpal tunnel syndrome (new onset or worsening) • Heel pain or plantar fasciitis • General body aches.

Cardiovascular Symptoms: • Heart palpitations (irregular heartbeat sensation) • Rapid heart rate (tachycardia) • Skipped heartbeats • Chest discomfort or pressure • Increased blood pressure • Increased cholesterol levels • Increased cardiovascular disease risk.

Skin, Hair & Nail Changes: • Dry skin • Itchy skin (pruritus)• Crawling or tingling skin sensations (formication) • Increased skin sensitivity • Thinning skin • Loss of skin elasticity • Increased wrinkles • Age spots or hyperpigmentation • Acne or adult acne • Rosacea (new onset or worsening) • Easy bruising • Hair thinning or loss (scalp) • Changes in hair texture • Increased facial hair growth (hirsutism) • Unwanted hair growth on chin or upper lip • Brittle nails • Ridged or splitting nails.

Gastrointestinal Symptoms: • Bloating • Gas and flatulence • Indigestion • Nausea • Constipation • Diarrhea • Changes in appetite • Weight gain (especially abdominal) • Difficulty losing weight • Food sensitivities or intolerances • irritable bowel syndrome (IBS) symptoms.

Breast Changes: • Breast tenderness or soreness • Breast swelling • Changes in breast size • Lumpy breasts (fibrocystic changes) • Nipple sensitivity.

Metabolic & Endocrine Changes: • Weight gain (particularly around midsection) • Changes in body fat distribution • Insulin resistance • Blood sugar fluctuations • Increased hunger or cravings • Thyroid dysfunction symptoms • Slowed metabolism • Difficulty maintaining weight.

Energy and Fatigue: • Chronic fatigue • Physical exhaustion • Mental exhaustion • Decreased stamina • Low energy levels • Weakness • Feeling of burnout.

Sensory Changes: • Dry eyes • Burning eyes • Vision changes (blurred vision) • Light sensitivity • Dry mouth • Altered sense of smell • Metallic taste in mouth • Electric shock sensations • Numbness or tingling in extremities • Increased sensitivity to pain.

Oral and Dental Changes: • Gum problems (bleeding, receding) • Tooth sensitivity • Dry mouth (xerostomia) • Burning mouth syndrome • Changes in taste • Increased dental cavities • Jaw pain or temporomandibular joint (TMJ) problems.

Respiratory Symptoms: • Asthma (new onset or worsening) • Allergies (new or worsening) • Sensation of breathlessness.

Body Odor and Temperature: • Changes in body odor • Changes in vaginal odor • Temperature regulation problems • Feeling too hot or too cold • Increased sweating.

Other Physical Symptoms: • Allergies (new or increased sensitivity) • Autoimmune condition flares • Inflammation (generalized) • Swelling or fluid retention • Restless leg syndrome • Leg cramps • Feeling of weakness in limbs.

The Variability You Need to Understand

One of the most frustrating aspects of this transition is how much variability exists between women:

Age of onset varies. Your mother's timeline does not predict yours. Your sister's experience will not match yours. Genetics play a role, but so do factors like smoking, nutrition, stress, autoimmune conditions, and previous pregnancies.

Symptom severity varies. About 20% of women breeze through with minimal symptoms. Another 20% suffer severely. Most fall somewhere in between. Why? We do not entirely know. Hormone receptor sensitivity, stress resilience, overall health, and genetic factors all contribute.

Duration varies. Some lucky women transition quickly, a couple of years from first irregular period to last period. Others spend a decade in the perimenopausal wilderness. Both are normal.

Symptom types vary. Your best friend might be debilitated by hot flashes while you barely notice them, but you are crippled by anxiety she never experiences. There are over 40 recognized symptoms of perimenopause and menopause. No one gets all of them. Most women experience a cluster of 5-10.

What Your Body Is Actually Doing

Let me explain the physiology in simple terms, because understanding what is happening helps it feel less frightening.

During your reproductive years, your ovaries contained thousands of follicles (fluid-filled sacs, each containing an egg). Every month, one follicle matured and released an egg, this is called ovulation. The follicle then transformed into the corpus luteum, which produced progesterone for the second half of your cycle. As you age, you have fewer follicles. The remaining ones become less responsive to the brain's hormonal signals (follicle stimulating hormone and luteinizing hormone, FSH and LH). Ovulation becomes sporadic. When you do not ovulate, you do not produce progesterone, but you often still produce estrogen.

This creates estrogen dominance: too much estrogen relative to progesterone. That is why many early perimenopausal symptoms, heavy bleeding, breast tenderness, bloating, and mood swings, mirror PMS (pre-menstrual syndrome) on steroids. Eventually, your ovaries produce less estrogen, but not smoothly. Some days estrogen surges. Other days it plummets. Your brain, sensing low estrogen, pumps out more FSH trying to stimulate your ovaries. This creates the hormonal rollercoaster that makes perimenopause so miserable.

Finally, your ovaries essentially retire. Estrogen and progesterone production drops to minimal levels. The chaos decreases. You have reached menopause.

The Most Important Takeaway

Here is what I want you to understand from this chapter:

Perimenopause is not menopause. If you are still having any periods, even if they are wildly irregular, you are in perimenopause, not menopause. This distinction matters for treatment.

The transition is a process, not an event. Just as you did not become a teenager overnight, you do not become postmenopausal overnight. This is a multi-year journey.

Normal is a wide range. Whatever you are experiencing, if it is not dangerous (we will cover warning signs in Chapter 3), is probably normal for you. But normal does not mean you have to suffer through it.

You do not have to wait until menopause to get help. So many women tough it out through perimenopause, thinking they will address symptoms "when I'm actually in menopause." But perimenopause is often when you need help most. Do not wait.

In the next chapter, we will dive deeper into the hormone shifts that drive these changes. Understanding the science will help you make informed decisions about treatment.

ACTION STEPS

1. **Identify which stage you are in** using the guidelines in this chapter.
2. **Track your menstrual patterns for 3 months** (even if irregular, noting dates and flow).
3. **Note when your symptoms started** relative to cycle changes.
4. **Remember: wherever you are in this journey is exactly where you are supposed to be.**

5. **Know that help is available at every stage** and you do not have to wait until you have reached menopause to seek treatment.

CHAPTER 2

The Hormone Shift - Your Body's Changing Chemistry

If you have ever felt like your body suddenly stopped following the rules, like someone changed the instruction manual without telling you, you are experiencing exactly what happens when your hormones shift during perimenopause and menopause. Understanding what is happening chemically inside your body is not just academic. When you know which hormones are declining and how that affects you, treatment options make more sense. You can have informed conversations with your healthcare provider. You can understand why certain symptoms cluster together. And perhaps most importantly, you can stop blaming yourself for what is a completely natural biological process.

The Four Key Hormones: Your Body's Chemical Messengers

Think of hormones as chemical messengers that travel through your bloodstream, delivering instructions to cells throughout your body. During your reproductive years, these messengers maintained predictable patterns. During perimenopause and menopause, those patterns change dramatically. Let us look at the four primary hormones involved in this transition:

ESTROGEN: The Master Regulator

What it does:

Estrogen is not just a "female hormone"; it is a whole-body regulator that affects virtually every system. Estrogen has about four-hundred (400) different functions in your body. During your reproductive years, your ovaries produced three types of estrogen:

estradiol (the most potent), estrone, and estriol. Estradiol was the dominant form.

Here is what estrogen influences:

Brain and Mood: Estrogen supports serotonin and dopamine production (your feel-good neurotransmitters). It affects memory, focus, and emotional regulation. This is why declining estrogen can trigger mood swings, anxiety, depression, and brain fog.

Temperature Regulation: Estrogen helps your hypothalamus (the brain's thermostat) maintain stable body temperature. When estrogen drops or fluctuates, your thermostat malfunctions, leading to the onset of, hot flashes and night sweats.

Sleep: Estrogen supports deep, restorative sleep. It also works with other neurotransmitters that regulate sleep-wake cycles. Lower estrogen often means worse sleep quality.

Bone Density: Estrogen inhibits bone breakdown and supports bone formation. When estrogen declines, bone loss accelerates dramatically, which is why osteoporosis risk increases after menopause.

Cardiovascular System: Estrogen keeps blood vessels flexible, supports healthy cholesterol levels, and protects against plaque formation. This is why heart disease risk increases after menopause.

Skin and Collagen: Estrogen stimulates collagen production, keeping skin elastic and hydrated. Less estrogen means thinner, drier skin and more wrinkles.

Vaginal and Urinary Health: Estrogen maintains the thickness and moisture of vaginal tissue and supports urinary tract health. Declining estrogen causes vaginal dryness, painful intercourse, and increased urinary tract infections.

Metabolism: Estrogen influences how your body stores and uses fat. When it declines, fat preferentially accumulates around your abdomen instead of hips and thighs.

What happens during perimenopause:

This is where it gets complicated. Estrogen levels do not decline smoothly. Instead, they fluctuate wildly, sometimes higher than ever, sometimes crashing to very low levels. You might have high estrogen one week (hello, sore breasts, and bloating) and low estrogen the next week leading to hot flashes and anxiety. These fluctuations are often more disruptive than the eventual low levels of post-menopause. It is the unpredictability that makes perimenopause so challenging.

What happens in post-menopause:

After your ovaries essentially stop producing estrogen, levels stabilize at a low baseline. Your adrenal glands and fat tissue produce small amounts of estrone (a weaker estrogen), but nothing like the estradiol of your reproductive years. For many women, once levels stabilize, some symptoms actually improve, even though estrogen remains low.

PROGESTERONE: The Calming Counterbalance

What it does:

If estrogen is the accelerator, progesterone is the brake. During your reproductive years, you produced progesterone during the second half of your menstrual cycle (after ovulation) from the corpus luteum, the transformed follicle that released the egg.

Here is what progesterone does:

Calming Effect: Progesterone metabolizes into allopregnanolone, which has anti-anxiety and sleep-promoting effects. It is nature's calming hormone.

Sleep Support: Progesterone enhances GABA (gamma-aminobutyric acid), a neurotransmitter that promotes deep, restorative sleep. This is why many women sleep better during the luteal phase of their cycle (when progesterone is high).

Mood Stabilization: Progesterone balances estrogen's effects on the brain and helps regulate mood.

Counterbalances Estrogen: Progesterone opposes many of estrogen's effects, preventing estrogen dominance symptoms like heavy bleeding, breast tenderness, and bloating.

Supports Pregnancy: In reproductive years, progesterone prepares the uterine lining for potential pregnancy and maintains early pregnancy.

Anti-Inflammatory: Progesterone has anti-inflammatory properties throughout the body.

What happens during perimenopause:

This is critical to understand: **progesterone often declines before estrogen does.**

Why? Because you only produce significant progesterone when you ovulate. As perimenopause progresses, ovulation becomes sporadic. You might skip ovulation multiple cycles in a row, which means multiple cycles with no progesterone production. Yet you are still producing estrogen. This creates **estrogen dominance**, not because estrogen is necessarily high, but because the estrogen-to-progesterone ratio is out of balance. This explains why many early perimenopausal symptoms mirror severe PMS (pre-menstrual syndrome):

- Heavy, prolonged menstrual bleeding
- Breast tenderness and swelling
- Bloating and water retention
- Mood swings and irritability
- Anxiety and insomnia
- Weight gain

Many women suffer with these symptoms for years without realizing that progesterone deficiency is the culprit.

What happens in post-menopause:

Once your ovaries stop functioning, progesterone production ceases almost entirely (you produce only trace amounts from your adrenal glands). For women who needed progesterone's calming effects, this can mean persistent anxiety and sleep problems, which is why progesterone supplementation can be so helpful even in post-menopause.

TESTOSTERONE: Not Just a Male Hormone

What it does:

Yes, women produce testosterone too, about one-tenth the amount men produce, but it is crucial nonetheless. Your ovaries and adrenal glands produce testosterone throughout your life.

Here is what testosterone does for women:

Energy and Vitality: Testosterone supports physical energy, motivation, and that general sense of "get up and go."

Muscle Mass and Strength: Testosterone helps build and maintain muscle tissue, which is crucial for metabolism and physical function.

Libido and Sexual Response: Testosterone is the primary hormone driving sexual desire, arousal, and satisfaction. It affects sensitivity and orgasm capacity.

Bone Strength: Like estrogen, testosterone supports bone density.

Mood and Confidence: Testosterone contributes to assertiveness, confidence, and mental sharpness.

Metabolism: Testosterone helps maintain lean muscle mass, which keeps your metabolism higher.

Cognitive Function: Testosterone supports memory, focus, and mental clarity.

What happens during perimenopause and menopause:

Testosterone levels begin declining in your 30s and continue dropping through perimenopause and menopause. However, the decline is more gradual than the dramatic shifts in estrogen and progesterone.

For some women, testosterone deficiency causes significant symptoms:

- Profound fatigue and lack of motivation
- Loss of libido (sometimes complete)
- Difficulty building or maintaining muscle despite exercise
- Decreased confidence and assertiveness
- Reduced mental sharpness
- Increased body fat despite no dietary changes

Many doctors overlook testosterone deficiency in women because they associate testosterone with men. But for women who are testosterone-deficient, replacing it can be transformative.

FSH and LH: The Brain's Desperate Signals

You will often hear about FSH (follicle-stimulating hormone) and LH (luteinizing hormone) in discussions about menopause. These hormones deserve a mention because they explain what your brain is doing during this transition.

What they do:

FSH and LH are produced by your pituitary gland (in your brain) to stimulate your ovaries. During your reproductive years, this system worked in elegant feedback loops: when estrogen was low, your brain released more FSH to stimulate your ovaries to produce estrogen. When estrogen was high enough, the brain reduced FSH.

What happens during perimenopause and menopause:

As your ovaries become less responsive, your brain detects low estrogen and pumps out more FSH and LH, desperately trying to get your ovaries to work harder. Your ovaries cannot comply because they are running out of follicles and declining in function.

The result? FSH and LH levels skyrocket. High FSH (typically over 25-30 IU/L, often reaching 100+ IU/L) is one marker that confirms you are approaching or have reached menopause. Some researchers believe these elevated FSH and LH levels contribute to symptoms like hot flashes, though this is still debated.

The Domino Effect: Why One Hormone Affects Everything

Now that you understand the individual hormones, let us look at how their decline creates a cascade of effects throughout your body.

The Brain: Lower estrogen and progesterone mean reduced serotonin, dopamine, and GABA, resulting in mood changes, anxiety, depression, brain fog, and poor sleep.

The Hypothalamus: Fluctuating estrogen disrupts temperature regulation, causing hot flashes and night sweats.

The Cardiovascular System: Lower estrogen means less flexible blood vessels, worse cholesterol profiles, and increased inflammation leads to rising heart disease risk.

The Bones: Lower estrogen means accelerated bone breakdown, increasing osteoporosis risk.

The Metabolism: Lower estrogen and testosterone mean less muscle mass, slower metabolic rate, and preferential abdominal fat storage, weight gain and body composition changes.

The Reproductive System: Lower estrogen means vaginal tissue thinning, dryness, and painful intercourse, which affects intimacy and quality of life.

The Urinary System: Lower estrogen means thinning urinary tract tissue, more infections and urgency.

The Skin: Lower estrogen means reduced collagen production—thinner, drier skin, more wrinkles.

Do you see how interconnected it all is? This is why menopause symptoms are not just about hot flashes. When your hormones shift, your entire body responds.

Estrogen Dominance vs. Estrogen Deficiency

This concept confuses many women, so let me clarify it because understanding this is crucial for treatment.

Estrogen Dominance occurs when you have too much estrogen relative to progesterone. This can happen because:

- Progesterone is very low (from lack of ovulation)
- Estrogen is normal or even high, but progesterone is missing

Symptoms of estrogen dominance:

- Heavy, prolonged menstrual bleeding
- Severe PMS symptoms
- Breast tenderness and swelling
- Bloating and water retention
- Mood swings and irritability
- Anxiety
- Weight gain, especially around hips and thighs
- Fibroids or endometriosis worsening

Estrogen Deficiency occurs when estrogen levels are truly low.

Symptoms of estrogen deficiency:

- Hot flashes and night sweats
- Vaginal dryness
- Insomnia
- Depression and anxiety
- Joint pain
- Dry skin and hair

- Low libido
- Urinary problems

Here is what makes perimenopause so confusing: You can experience both patterns, sometimes even in the same month. One week you might be estrogen dominant (sore breasts, bloating). The next week you crash into estrogen deficiency (hot flashes, insomnia).

This is why perimenopausal treatment often requires both progesterone (to balance excess estrogen) and sometimes estrogen (during the crashes). It is not one-size-fits-all.

Why Hormone Testing Can Be Misleading

Many women ask: "Can I just test my hormones to see what is happening?"

The answer is: it is complicated.

In perimenopause, hormone testing is notoriously unreliable. Why? Because your levels fluctuate dramatically from day to day, even hour to hour. A test showing low estrogen on Monday might show high estrogen on Wednesday. The snapshot test provided does not capture the chaos.

That said, testing can sometimes be useful to:

- Rule out other conditions (thyroid problems, for example)
- Assess whether you have reached menopause (very high FSH suggests you have)
- Monitor hormone therapy (to ensure levels are appropriate)

In post-menopause, testing is more reliable because levels are more stable.

The bottom line: Diagnosis and treatment of perimenopausal and menopausal symptoms should be based primarily on your symptoms and menstrual pattern, not hormone levels. An experienced provider will listen to what you are experiencing and treat accordingly.

The Good News About Understanding Your Hormones

Now that you understand what is happening chemically, several things should make more sense:

Your symptoms are real and biological. You are not crazy. You are not weak. You are not imagining things. Your hormones are changing, and your body is responding exactly as it should to those changes.

Different symptoms respond to different treatments. If you are progesterone-deficient, adding estrogen will not fully help. If you are testosterone-deficient, estrogen and progesterone will not restore your energy and libido. Matching treatment to your specific hormone deficiencies is key.

Timing matters. What you need in early perimenopause (perhaps progesterone for estrogen dominance) may differ from what you need in late perimenopause or post-menopause (perhaps estrogen and progesterone together).

Lifestyle affects hormones. While you cannot stop the natural decline, your nutrition, exercise, stress management, and sleep quality influence how your body responds to hormonal changes. We will cover this in detail in Chapter 7.

You have options. Now that you understand the hormones involved, you can appreciate why bioidentical hormone replacement can be so effective, as you are literally replacing what your body is no longer producing. But you also have other options: nutraceuticals that support your body's remaining hormone production or help you better utilize the hormones you still have, and lifestyle strategies that optimize your hormonal environment.

Moving Forward

In the next chapter, we will discuss the full spectrum of symptoms you might experience during this transition. Some will be obvious. Others might be surprising, you may not have realized they were related to hormones at all.

But now you have the basics. You understand that perimenopause and menopause are not mysterious or vague conditions. They are specific, biological processes involving measurable hormones affecting every system in your body.

And because they are biological, they are treatable.

ACTION STEPS

1. **Review the hormone descriptions** and identify which symptoms match your experience.
2. **Notice patterns:** Do your symptoms correlate with your menstrual cycle? This can reveal whether progesterone deficiency is playing a role.
3. **Consider whether you might be experiencing estrogen dominance, estrogen deficiency, or both at different times**.
4. **Remember that testosterone deficiency is real in women** and can explain persistent fatigue and low libido that does not respond to estrogen and progesterone alone.
5. **Do not rely solely on hormone testing to diagnose perimenopause**, your symptoms and cycle pattern are more informative.
6. **Keep a symptom journal for 2-4 weeks** noting what you experience and when—this will be invaluable when talking to your healthcare provider.

CHAPTER 3

The Signs and Symptoms - Recognizing What Is Happening

When I ask women in my practice what symptoms they are experiencing, most start with the obvious ones: hot flashes, irregular periods, maybe some trouble sleeping. But when I hand them a comprehensive symptom checklist, their eyes widen.

"Wait? The joint pain is from perimenopause?"

"I thought the brain fog meant I was developing dementia."

"Nobody told me that anxiety could be hormonal."

"My hair loss is connected to THIS?"

There are over 40 recognized symptoms associated with perimenopause and menopause. No woman experiences all of them. Most experience a cluster of 5-15. But recognizing which symptoms are hormone-related is the first step toward getting appropriate treatment.

In this chapter, we will walk through most of symptoms—from the well-known to the surprising. As you read, I encourage you to check off which ones you are experiencing. This will give you a clear picture to share with your healthcare provider.

The Classic Trio: What Everyone Knows About

Let us start with the symptoms most commonly associated with menopause:

Hot Flashes (Vasomotor Symptoms)

What they feel like: A sudden sensation of intense heat, usually starting in your chest or face and spreading through your upper body. Your skin may flush red. Your heart may race. You might sweat profusely. The episode typically lasts 1-5 minutes but can feel eternal.

How common: About 75-85% of women experience hot flashes during perimenopause or menopause. For about 10-15% of women, they are severe enough to significantly impact quality of life.

When they occur: Hot flashes can begin in early perimenopause and continue for years. Some women experience them for only a year or two. Others deal with them for a decade or more. The average duration is 7-10 years.

What causes them: Fluctuating or declining estrogen disrupts your hypothalamus (the brain's temperature control center), causing it to mistakenly perceive that your body is overheating. The body then tries to cool itself down with profuse sweating, and vasodilation (blood vessel expansion) as it tries to release the heat from surface blood vessels.

Impact: Beyond physical discomfort, hot flashes can be embarrassing (particularly at work or in social situations), disruptive (waking you multiple times per night), and exhausting (the adrenaline surge leaves you depleted).

Night Sweats

What they feel like: Hot flashes that occur during sleep, often drenching your sheets, pillows, and nightclothes. You might wake up soaked, chilled from the evaporating sweat, and need to change clothes or bedding.

How common: About 75% of women with hot flashes also experience night sweats.

Impact: Night sweats are particularly problematic because they fragment your sleep. Even if you fall back asleep quickly, your sleep architecture is disrupted. You miss out on deep, restorative sleep stages. Over time, this leads to severe sleep deprivation with cascading effects on mood, cognition, energy, and health.

Irregular Periods

What they look like: Your previously predictable menstrual cycle becomes unpredictable. Periods might come every 21 days, then skip two months, then arrive again. Flow might be lighter than normal, then suddenly much heavier. Duration might change from your typical 5 days, to 2 days or 10 days.

How common: Nearly 100% of women in perimenopause experience menstrual irregularity at some point.

When to be concerned: While irregular periods are normal in perimenopause, certain patterns warrant medical evaluation:

- Bleeding after 12 months without a period (this is never normal)
- Extremely heavy bleeding (soaking through a pad or tampon every hour)
- Bleeding lasting more than 7-10 days
- Bleeding after intercourse
- Bleeding between periods

These patterns could indicate fibroids, polyps, endometrial hyperplasia, or rarely, more serious conditions. Always report them to your healthcare provider.

Sleep Disturbances: More Than Just Night Sweats

Many women assume their sleep problems are solely from night sweats. But hormonal changes affect sleep in multiple ways:

Difficulty Falling Asleep

What it feels like: You are exhausted, you go to bed, but your mind races. You cannot shut off your thoughts. You lie awake for 30 minutes, an hour, sometimes longer.

What causes it: Low progesterone reduces GABA (the calming neurotransmitter), making it harder to transition from wakefulness to sleep. Low estrogen affects serotonin, which also influences sleep initiation.

Difficulty Staying Asleep

What it feels like: You fall asleep fine but wake at 2 or 3 or 4 AM, wide awake, mind racing. Sometimes you fall back asleep after an hour. Sometimes you do not.

What causes it: Hormonal fluctuations, particularly the cortisol-progesterone imbalance. Declining progesterone fails to suppress your stress response adequately, allowing cortisol spikes that wake you in the early morning hours.

Non-Restorative Sleep

What it feels like: You sleep for 7-8 hours but wake feeling like you never slept at all. You are exhausted all day despite adequate time in bed.

What causes it: Disrupted sleep architecture. Even without full awakenings, hormonal changes can prevent you from reaching deep sleep stages or cause frequent micro-arousals you do not consciously remember.

Impact: Chronic poor sleep affects everything: mood, cognition, metabolism, immune function, pain perception, and cardiovascular health. Addressing sleep is not optional, klit is foundational to feeling better.

Mood and Emotional Changes: Not "All in Your Head"

This is where many women feel most gaslit. Doctors minimize these symptoms. Partners do not understand. You start questioning your sanity.

Let me be clear: **these symptoms are real, biological, and hormone-related.**

Mood Swings

What they feel like: Emotional volatility that feels out of proportion to the situation. You are fine one moment and crying the next. Small frustrations trigger disproportionate anger. You feel like you are on an emotional rollercoaster.

What causes them: Fluctuating estrogen and progesterone directly affect neurotransmitter levels (serotonin, dopamine, GABA). When hormones swing wildly, your emotions often do the same.

Anxiety

What it feels like: Free-floating worry that was not there before. Racing heart. Sense of impending doom. Panic attacks. Catastrophic thinking. Social anxiety you never previously experienced.

What causes it: Low progesterone reduces your brain's GABA (the anti-anxiety neurotransmitter). Low estrogen affects serotonin, which regulates anxiety. The result is a chemically induced anxiety state.

Important distinction: This is not the same as having an anxiety disorder, though it can feel identical. This is hormonally driven anxiety that often responds beautifully to hormone restoration.

Depression

What it feels like: Persistent sadness, hopelessness, loss of interest in activities you once enjoyed, difficulty feeling pleasure, crying spells, a sense of emptiness.

What causes it: Declining estrogen reduces serotonin production and sensitivity. The risk of depression doubles during perimenopause compared to premenopausal years.

Important: If you have a history of depression, perimenopause can trigger recurrence even if you have been stable for years. If you are having thoughts of self-harm, seek help immediately. Hormone-related depression is treatable, but it is also serious.

Irritability and Rage

What it feels like: A short fuse. Snapping at loved ones. Road rage. Explosive anger over minor irritations. Afterward, you feel guilty and wonder what is wrong with you.

What causes it: The combination of poor sleep, fluctuating serotonin, low progesterone, and physiological stress from other symptoms creates a perfect storm for irritability.

Cognitive Changes: The "Fuzzy Brain" Phenomenon

This cluster of symptoms terrifies many women because they fear dementia or Alzheimer's disease.

Brain Fog

What it feels like: Mental cloudiness, like thinking through cotton wool. Difficulty concentrating. Trouble following conversations or reading comprehension. A general sense that your brain is not working properly.

What causes it: Estrogen is crucial for brain metabolism and neurotransmitter function. When it fluctuates or declines, cognitive function suffers temporarily.

Memory Problems

What they look like: Forgetting words mid-sentence. Walking into a room and forgetting why. Losing your keys repeatedly. Forgetting appointments or names. Short-term memory feels unreliable.

What causes them: Estrogen influences the hippocampus (memory center) and supports acetylcholine (memory neurotransmitter). Lower estrogen temporarily impairs memory formation and retrieval.

Reassurance: For most women, these cognitive changes are temporary and improve with hormone stabilization or treatment. This is not dementia. Your brain is not degenerating. It is responding to hormonal fluctuations, and function typically returns.

Difficulty with Words

What it feels like: You know what you want to say but cannot find the word. You describe things instead of naming them. You substitute incorrect words and catch yourself afterward.

What causes it: Estrogen influences language centers in the brain. Fluctuations disrupt word retrieval pathways.

Physical Changes: Your Body Feels Different

Beyond the obvious reproductive changes, perimenopause and menopause cause numerous physical symptoms:

Weight Gain and Body Composition Changes

What it looks like: Weight creeping up despite no changes in diet or exercise. Fat redistributing to your abdomen instead of hips and thighs. Losing muscle tone even if you are exercising.

What causes it: Declining estrogen and testosterone reduce muscle mass and slow metabolism. Estrogen loss causes preferential abdominal fat storage. Insulin sensitivity decreases, making weight loss harder.

Average: Women gain 5-15 pounds during the menopausal transition, with significant increases in visceral (abdominal) fat.

Joint and Muscle Pain

What it feels like: Aching joints, particularly in hands, knees, and shoulders. Morning stiffness. Generalized muscle aches. Some women develop frozen shoulder or trigger finger.

What causes it: Estrogen has anti-inflammatory properties. When it declines, inflammation increases, affecting joints and connective tissue.

Fatigue

What it feels like: Bone-deep exhaustion not relieved by rest. Lack of physical energy. Difficulty getting through basic daily tasks.

What causes it: Poor sleep, low thyroid function (which often declines concurrently), low testosterone, anemia from heavy bleeding, depression, and the simple physiological stress of hormonal chaos.

Headaches and Migraines

What they look like: New-onset headaches or worsening of existing migraine patterns. Headaches that correlate with your menstrual cycle.

What causes them: Estrogen withdrawal triggers migraines in susceptible women. The hormonal fluctuations of perimenopause can dramatically worsen migraine frequency and severity.

Breast Tenderness and Changes

What it feels like: Sore, swollen breasts. Increased lumpiness (fibrocystic changes). Sensitivity that makes even wearing a bra uncomfortable.

What causes it: Estrogen dominance (high estrogen relative to progesterone) stimulates breast tissue. This is particularly common in early perimenopause.

Heart Palpitations

What they feel like: Awareness of your heartbeat. Feeling like your heart is racing, pounding, or skipping beats. Sometimes accompanied by anxiety or chest discomfort.

What causes them: Declining estrogen affects the autonomic nervous system and can trigger palpitations. They are usually benign but always warrant cardiac evaluation to rule out actual heart problems.

Dizziness and Vertigo

What it feels like: Lightheadedness, spinning sensations, balance problems, feeling like you might faint.

What causes it: Blood pressure changes from vasomotor symptoms, inner ear changes from hormone fluctuations, and sometimes related to anxiety or panic.

Changes in Sexual Health and Intimacy

These symptoms profoundly affect quality of life and relationships but often go unaddressed because women feel embarrassed to discuss them.

Low Libido (Decreased Sexual Desire)

What it feels like: You simply do not think about sex anymore. You are not interested. You might agree to sex for your partner's sake, but you feel no desire yourself.

What causes it: Declining testosterone (the primary libido hormone), low estrogen affecting arousal, progesterone causing sedation, physical discomfort from vaginal changes, and the psychological impact of other symptoms.

Vaginal Dryness

What it feels like: Lack of natural lubrication. Discomfort or burning sensation in the vaginal area. Sometimes itching or irritation.

What causes it: Declining estrogen causes vaginal tissue to thin (vaginal atrophy), lose elasticity, and produce less moisture. This condition, called genitourinary syndrome of menopause (GSM), affects up to 50-70% of postmenopausal women.

Painful Intercourse (Dyspareunia)

What it feels like: Sex hurts. Penetration is uncomfortable or painful. You might experience tearing, burning, or bleeding afterward.

What causes it: Vaginal atrophy from low estrogen combined with decreased lubrication. Vaginal tissue becomes fragile and less elastic.

Impact: Many women avoid intimacy because of pain, which strains relationships. Partners may feel rejected. Women feel guilty and broken. But this is eminently treatable.

Decreased Arousal and Difficulty with Orgasm

What it feels like: Even when you want to be intimate, your body does not respond the way it used to. Arousal takes longer. Orgasms are harder to achieve or less intense.

What causes it: Decreased blood flow to genital tissues from low estrogen and testosterone. Reduced nerve sensitivity. Thinning tissue with fewer nerve endings.

Hair, Skin, and Nail Changes

Estrogen influences your body's largest organ, which is your skin, as well as hair and nails.

Hair Loss and Thinning

What it looks like: More hair in your brush or shower drain. Widening part line. Thinning at the temples. Overall decrease in hair volume and thickness.

What causes it: Declining estrogen (which supports hair growth) combined with relatively higher androgens (male hormones) shifts the ratio, triggering hair thinning or loss. Some women also lose eyebrows or eyelashes.

Dry Skin

What it feels like: Skin that feels tight, rough, and uncomfortable. Loss of that youthful plumpness. Increased itching.

What causes it: Estrogen stimulates oil glands and collagen production. Without it, skin becomes drier and thinner.

Increased Wrinkles

What it looks like: Accelerated aging of facial skin. Fine lines becoming deeper. Loss of elasticity and firmness.

What causes it: Collagen production drops by about 30% in the first five years after menopause. Without collagen, skin loses its structural support.

Brittle Nails

What they look like: Nails that split, peel, or break easily. Ridges developing. Slower growth.

What causes them: Declining estrogen affects keratin production and nail bed health.

Urinary Changes

These symptoms are common but rarely discussed.

Urinary Urgency and Frequency

What it feels like: Sudden, intense need to urinate with little warning. Needing to urinate more frequently, including multiple times per night.

What causes it: Declining estrogen affects bladder and urethral tissue, reducing capacity and increasing sensitivity.

Stress Incontinence

What it looks like: Leaking urine when you cough, sneeze, laugh, or exercise.

What causes it: Weakening of pelvic floor muscles and tissues that support the bladder, partially from declining estrogen.

Recurrent Urinary Tract Infections

What they are: More frequent bladder infections than you experienced previously.

What causes them: Thinning urethral tissue and changes in vaginal pH from declining estrogen make you more susceptible to infections.

The Surprising Symptoms: Things You Never Expected

These symptoms often surprise women because they seem unrelated to hormones:

Burning Mouth or Tongue

What it feels like: A burning, scalding sensation in your mouth, tongue, or throat without visible cause.

What causes it: Changes in nerve function and decreased saliva production from declining estrogen.

Tingling in Extremities

What it feels like: Numbness, tingling, or "pins and needles" sensations in hands, feet, arms, or legs.

What causes it: Hormonal effects on nerve function, circulation, and sometimes B vitamin deficiency.

Electric Shock Sensations

What they feel like: Brief, sudden jolts or zaps, often in the head or before a hot flash.

What causes them: Neurological effects of estrogen fluctuation on nerve fibers.

Changes in Taste and Smell

What it is like: Foods tasting different than they used to. Decreased sense of smell. Metallic taste in your mouth.

What causes it: Hormonal influences on taste buds and olfactory receptors.

Digestive Changes

What it looks like: New food sensitivities. Bloating that was not there before. Changes in bowel habits. Increased gas.

What causes it: Estrogen affects gut motility and the gut microbiome. Progesterone slows digestion.

Allergies and Sensitivities

What it looks like: Developing new allergies or sensitivities to foods, environmental triggers, or substances you previously tolerated.

What causes it: Hormonal influences on immune function and histamine response.

When Symptoms Signal Something More Serious

While most perimenopausal and menopausal symptoms are benign, certain red flags warrant immediate medical evaluation:

Seek urgent care if you experience:

- Chest pain or pressure (rule out heart problems)
- Severe headache unlike any you have had before (rule out stroke)
- Visual changes or loss of vision (rule out stroke or retinal problems)
- Confusion or difficulty speaking (rule out stroke)
- Severe abdominal pain (rule out ovarian or other abdominal pathology)

- Bleeding after 12 months without a period (rule out endometrial hyperplasia or cancer)
- Extremely heavy bleeding (soaking through protection hourly) or passing large clots

Schedule an appointment soon if you experience:

- Suicidal thoughts or severe depression
- Severe anxiety or panic attacks affecting function
- Palpitations, especially if associated with chest discomfort or shortness of breath
- Persistent digestive symptoms (rule out gallbladder, gastrointestinal conditions)
- Unexplained weight loss
- Severe fatigue despite adequate rest (rule out thyroid, anemia, other conditions)

Many conditions can mimic or co-occur with perimenopause: thyroid disorders, anemia, diabetes, autoimmune conditions, depression, and anxiety disorders. Your healthcare provider needs to rule these out.

You Are Not Imagining This

If you checked off multiple symptoms while reading this chapter, you might feel overwhelmed. That is normal. But here is what I want you to know:

Every symptom you are experiencing is real. You are not being dramatic. You are not weak. You are not imagining things. Your body is responding to profound hormonal shifts, and those shifts create measurable, biological symptoms.

You are not alone. Millions of women worldwide are experiencing exactly what you are experiencing. The symptoms vary in severity and combination, but the process is universal.

Most importantly: you do not have to suffer through this. Every symptom we discussed in this chapter is treatable. Some respond to hormone therapy. Others respond to nutraceuticals, lifestyle changes, or non-hormonal medications. Many respond to a combination.

In the next section of this handbook, we will explore all your treatment options, from bioidentical hormones to physician-grade supplements to lifestyle strategies. You will learn how to address each symptom cluster along with your healthcare provider, and create a personalized plan that works for you.

But first, take a moment to acknowledge what you are going through. Validate your experience. And recognize that seeking help is not weakness, it is wisdom.

ACTION STEPS

1. **Review the symptom list** and check off what you are experiencing.
2. **Rate each symptom's severity** (mild, moderate, severe) and how much it affects your daily life.
3. **Note when symptoms started** and whether they correlate with menstrual cycle changes.
4. **Identify your top 3-5 most disruptive symptoms**, these become your treatment priorities.
5. **Rule out red flag symptoms** that need immediate medical evaluation.
6. **Share this information with your healthcare provider**, bring your symptom list to appointments.
7. **Remember: recognizing what is happening is the first step toward feeling better**.

"I had many of the symptoms on that list. Sixteen. And I was just trying to power through, thinking this was normal aging. Once I realized it was all connected to perimenopause, I finally got treatment. Within three months, I felt like myself again."

— Linda, 48, Canada

PART II

YOUR INTEGRATIVE TREATMENT OPTIONS

CHAPTER 4

Bioidentical Hormone Replacement Therapy (BHRT) - The Evidence-Based Truth

Few topics in women's health generate as much confusion, conflicting information, and fear as hormone replacement therapy. You have probably heard terrifying warnings about cancer risk. You have probably also heard miraculous success stories from women who swear hormones saved their lives.

Both perspectives contain elements of truth, but neither tells the complete story.

As a physician who prescribes bioidentical hormones and who takes them myself, I want to give you accurate, evidence-based information so you can make an informed decision. No hype. No fear-mongering. Just facts.

Let us start by clarifying what we are actually talking about.

HRT vs. BHRT: Understanding the Difference

The terms HRT (Hormone Replacement Therapy) and BHRT (Bioidentical Hormone Replacement Therapy) are often used interchangeably, but there are important distinctions.

Traditional HRT (Conventional Hormone Replacement Therapy)

What it is: Traditional HRT typically refers to synthetic or animal-derived hormones that are not molecularly identical to the hormones your body produces naturally.

Common examples:

- **Premarin** (conjugated equine estrogens, derived from pregnant mare's urine)
- **Provera** (medroxyprogesterone acetate, a synthetic form of progesterone)
- **Prempro** (combination of Premarin and Provera)

How it differs from your natural hormones:

Traditional HRT uses hormones that are chemically different from what your body makes. Premarin contains horse estrogens (equilin and equilenin) that are foreign to the human body. Provera is a synthetic progestin; it is not natural progesterone. It has a different molecular structure that creates different effects in your body.

Your body has receptors designed for human estradiol and progesterone. When you give it horse estrogens or synthetic progestins, these molecules fit into the receptors differently, like using a key that works but does not fit perfectly. This can create side effects and potentially different health outcomes.

The WHI Study and why it matters:

In the 2002 Women's Health Initiative (WHI) study, the one that terrified millions of women away from hormones, they studied Prempro (Premarin plus Provera). It found increased risks of breast cancer, heart disease, stroke, and blood clots in women taking this particular combination.

This study was important, but here is what most people do not understand: **The risks identified were specifically associated with oral conjugated equine estrogens plus synthetic progestins, not with bioidentical hormones.**

The study did not evaluate bioidentical estradiol or natural progesterone. Yet the findings were broadly applied to ALL hormone therapy, creating decades of confusion and fear.

Bioidentical Hormone Replacement Therapy (BHRT)

What it is: BHRT uses hormones that are molecularly identical to the ones your body produces naturally. The chemical structure is the same as human estradiol, progesterone, and testosterone.

Where it comes from: Despite being "bioidentical" to human hormones, these hormones are not extracted from humans. They are synthesized in laboratories from plant sources (typically soy or yam). Through a chemical process, the plant compounds are converted into molecules identical to human hormones.

How it works in your body: Because bioidentical hormones have precisely the same molecular structure as your natural hormones, they fit perfectly into your hormone receptors. Your body recognizes them as its own and processes them the same way it would your naturally produced hormones.

Forms of bioidentical hormones:

FDA-Approved Bioidentical Hormones:

- **Estradiol:** Available as pills, patches, gels, creams, vaginal tablets, and vaginal rings (brands include Estrace, Climara, Vivelle-Dot, Divigel, EstroGel, Vagifem)
- **Progesterone:** Available as oral capsules and vaginal gel (brands include Prometrium, Crinone)
- **Testosterone:** Available as pellets, gels, and creams (though fewer FDA-approved options exist specifically for women)

Compounded Bioidentical Hormones: We will discuss these in detail shortly, but these are custom-formulated by specialized pharmacies.

Key distinction: Just because a hormone is FDA-approved does not mean it is not bioidentical, and just because it is compounded does not automatically make it bioidentical. What matters is the molecular structure. Bioidentical means molecularly identical to human hormones, regardless of whether it is FDA-approved or compounded.

Why the Distinction Matters for Your Health

Research has increasingly shown that **bioidentical hormones, particularly transdermal (through the skin) estradiol combined with oral micronized progesterone, have a different safety profile than traditional synthetic HRT.**

Studies indicate that:

- Bioidentical progesterone does not increase breast cancer risk the way synthetic progestins do
- Transdermal estradiol has lower blood clot risk than oral estrogen
- Bioidentical hormones more closely mimic natural hormonal patterns
- Side effects tend to be fewer and milder with bioidentical hormones

This is why, as a physician, I prescribe bioidentical hormones almost exclusively. The risk-benefit profile is more favorable, and patient outcomes are typically better.

FDA-Approved BHRT vs. Compounded BHRT

Now that you understand what bioidentical means, let us discuss another important distinction: FDA-approved versus compounded bioidentical hormones.

FDA-Approved Bioidentical Hormones

What they are: These are commercially manufactured bioidentical hormones that have undergone FDA approval processes. They are mass-produced in standardized doses by pharmaceutical companies.

Advantages:

- Extensively studied and regulated
- Consistent dosing and quality control
- Insurance coverage is more likely
- Long track record of safety and efficacy

- Widely available at most pharmacies

Limitations:

- Fixed doses (cannot be as easily customized)
- Limited delivery methods for some hormones
- May contain fillers or additives that some women react to
- Not all combinations are available in single products

Examples:

- **Estradiol patches** (Climara, Vivelle-Dot): deliver steady estradiol through skin
- **Estradiol gels** (Estrogel, Divigel): applied daily to skin
- **Oral micronized progesterone** (Prometrium): capsules taken at night
- **Vaginal estradiol** (Vagifem, Imvexxy): tablets or inserts for local treatment

Many women do beautifully with FDA-approved bioidentical hormones. They are my first choice for most patients because of the extensive safety data and quality assurance.

Compounded Bioidentical Hormones

What they are: Custom-formulated hormone preparations made by specialized compounding pharmacies according to a healthcare provider's prescription. These can combine multiple hormones, adjust doses precisely, and use different delivery methods.

How compounding works:

A compounding pharmacy is not just filling prescriptions, it is creating customized medications. The pharmacist starts with pharmaceutical-grade bioidentical hormones (the same raw materials used by commercial manufacturers) and compounds them into specific formulations based on your provider's prescription.

Advantages:

Customization: Doses can be adjusted in tiny increments to match your specific needs. If you need 0.75 mg of estradiol (a dose not commercially available), a compounding pharmacy can make it.

Combination products: Multiple hormones can be combined into a single cream or capsule. For example, estradiol, progesterone, and testosterone in one topical cream, rather than using three separate products.

Alternative delivery methods: Compounding allows for formulations not commercially available, such as:

- Sublingual troches (dissolve under tongue)
- Topical creams with specific absorption bases
- Vaginal suppositories with customized combinations
- Slow-release capsules

Allergen avoidance: Compounding pharmacies can create formulations without specific fillers, dyes, gluten, or other ingredients that cause reactions in sensitive patients.

Hormone variety: Compounders can include hormones not easily available commercially, such as DHEA, pregnenolone, or specific estrogen ratios (Biest—80% estriol/20% estradiol, or Triest—80% estriol/10% estradiol/10% estrone).

When compounded BHRT makes sense:

- Standard doses are too high or too low for your needs
- You need a hormone combination not commercially available
- You are sensitive to fillers in commercial products
- You want to minimize the number of products you use daily
- Your provider prefers specific formulations based on clinical experience
- You need access to hormones not widely available in commercial form

Considerations and limitations:

Quality varies: Not all compounding pharmacies are equal. Quality control, purity testing, and consistency can vary. It is crucial to use a reputable compounding pharmacy that follows USP (United States Pharmacopeia) standards and regularly tests their products.

Less research: While the bioidentical hormones themselves are well-studied, specific compounded formulations may not have the same extensive research as FDA-approved products.

Cost: Compounded hormones are often not covered by insurance, making them more expensive out-of-pocket.

Absorption variability: Some compounded formulations (particularly creams) can have variable absorption rates between individuals. What works for one woman may not deliver consistent levels for another.

Regulatory differences: Compounded hormones are not FDA-approved (though the raw hormones used are typically pharmaceutical-grade). The FDA regulates compounding pharmacies but differently than commercial manufacturers.

Finding reputable compounding pharmacies:

If you and your provider decide compounded hormones are right for you, choose a pharmacy that:

- Is accredited by the Pharmacy Compounding Accreditation Board (PCAB)
- Follows USP guidelines
- Provides certificates of analysis for hormone potency
- Has a good reputation among experienced hormone prescribers
- Communicates clearly about their quality control processes

My Approach as a Prescriber

I use both FDA-approved and compounded bioidentical hormones depending on the patient's needs:

I start with FDA-approved bioidentical hormones when:

- The patient has straightforward needs that standard doses address
- Cost is a concern (insurance coverage helps)
- The patient prefers the security of FDA-approved products
- Standard formulations are working well

I use compounded bioidentical hormones when:

- Standard doses do not work (too high or too low)
- The patient needs a combination product for convenience
- The patient has sensitivities to commercial fillers
- We need very precise dose adjustments
- The patient specifically requests compounded formulations

Both approaches use bioidentical hormones. Both can be highly effective. The choice depends on your individual situation, preferences, and what your body responds to best.

What BHRT Actually Does: The Benefits

Now let us talk about what bioidentical hormone replacement can do for you when properly prescribed.

Relief of Vasomotor Symptoms

Hot flashes and night sweats: Estrogen is the single most effective treatment for hot flashes, with 80-90% reduction in frequency and severity for most women. Estrogen comes in Synthetic, Bioidentical and Phytomedicines. Discussion with your healthcare provider to assist you with the best choice for you is important.

Timeline: Most women notice improvement within 2-4 weeks, with maximum benefit by 3 months.

Improved Sleep

Multiple mechanisms: Estrogen and progesterone both support sleep through different pathways. Estrogen improves sleep quality and reduces night sweats that fragment sleep. Progesterone has sedating properties that help you fall asleep and stay asleep.

Timeline: Sleep often improves within 1-2 weeks of starting progesterone, sometimes immediately. Estrogen's effects on sleep through reduced night sweats take 2-4 weeks.

Mood Stabilization

Anxiety and depression: For hormonally driven mood changes, estrogen and progesterone can be remarkably effective. Estrogen supports serotonin production. Progesterone enhances GABA (the calming neurotransmitter).

Timeline: Mood improvements typically begin within 2-4 weeks and continue improving over 2-3 months.

Important: BHRT is not a substitute for treatment of clinical depression or anxiety disorders, but for hormonally driven mood symptoms, it can be transformative.

Cognitive Function

Brain fog and memory: Estrogen is crucial for brain metabolism and neurotransmitter function. Women often report improved mental clarity, better memory, and sharper focus on BHRT.

Timeline: Cognitive improvements usually become noticeable within 4-8 weeks.

Vaginal and Urinary Health

Vaginal atrophy: Estrogen, particularly when applied locally as a cream, tablet, or ring, reverses vaginal thinning, restores moisture, improves elasticity, and eliminates painful intercourse.

Urinary symptoms: Vaginal estrogen also improves urinary symptoms like urgency, frequency, and recurrent infections.

Timeline: Vaginal symptoms typically improve within 2-4 weeks of starting vaginal estrogen, with continued improvement over 3 months.

Sexual Function

Libido: Testosterone is the primary hormone for sexual desire. Many women experience restored libido with testosterone replacement. Estrogen also helps by improving vaginal health and reducing pain.

Timeline: Libido improvements with testosterone typically take 6-12 weeks to become noticeable.

Bone Density Protection

Osteoporosis prevention: Estrogen is one of the most effective treatments for preventing bone loss. It inhibits osteoclasts (cells that break down bone) and supports osteoblasts (cells that build bone).

Research shows: Women on BHRT maintain significantly better bone density than untreated women and have reduced fracture risk.

Cardiovascular Protection

Heart health: When started during perimenopause or early menopause (before age 60 or within 10 years of final period), estrogen has cardiovascular benefits: improved cholesterol profiles, better vascular function, and reduced plaque formation.

Important timing: This benefit appears to be time-sensitive. Starting hormones early in the transition offers cardiovascular protection. Starting after age 60 or more than 10 years past menopause may not offer the same benefit and could increase risk.

Metabolic Benefits

Body composition: BHRT (Bioidentical hormone replacement therapy), particularly when including testosterone, helps maintain muscle mass and can improve body composition. Some women find it easier to manage weight on hormones.

Insulin sensitivity: Estrogen improves insulin sensitivity, which supports metabolic health.

Skin, Hair, and Overall Vitality

Skin quality: Estrogen stimulates collagen production, improves skin thickness, and enhances moisture. Many women notice improved skin quality on BHRT.

Hair: While BHRT cannot fully prevent age-related hair thinning, it can slow the process and improve hair thickness.

Energy and vitality: This is harder to quantify, but countless women report feeling "like myself again". They report more energy, more vitality, better mood, clearer thinking. The cumulative effect of improved sleep, stable mood, better cognition, and physical comfort is profound.

Who Benefits Most from BHRT

BHRT is not right for everyone, but many women are excellent candidates.

You may be an ideal candidate if:

- You have moderate to severe menopausal symptoms affecting quality of life
- Your symptoms started in perimenopause or early menopause

- You want the most effective treatment for hot flashes and night sweats
- You have vaginal atrophy causing painful intercourse
- You have osteoporosis or significant bone loss
- You are within 10 years of your final period and under age 60
- You have no contraindications (we will discuss these shortly)
- You want to optimize long-term health (bone, heart, brain)

BHRT can be particularly beneficial for women with:

- Surgical menopause (ovaries removed)
- Premature or early menopause (before age 45)
- Severe perimenopausal symptoms
- Strong family history of osteoporosis
- Testosterone deficiency symptoms (low libido, fatigue, loss of muscle)

Who Should Avoid BHRT or Use It with Caution

Certain conditions make hormone therapy inappropriate or require special consideration:

Absolute contraindications (you should NOT take systemic estrogen):

- History of breast cancer (with rare exceptions and specialized care)
- History of estrogen-receptor positive cancers
- Active or recent blood clots (deep vein thrombosis-DVT or pulmonary embolism)
- History of stroke
- Unexplained vaginal bleeding
- Active liver disease
- Known or suspected pregnancy

Relative contraindications (proceed with caution, specialist input):

- Personal history of blood clotting disorders

- Strong family history of blood clots
- History of heart disease
- Migraine with aura (increased stroke risk)
- Gallbladder disease
- High triglycerides
- Fibroids or endometriosis (may worsen with estrogen)

Important note about breast cancer: While systemic estrogen is contraindicated in most breast cancer survivors, *vaginal estrogen for treating vaginal atrophy is often considered safe* even in this population because it is absorbed minimally and does not significantly raise blood estrogen levels. This decision should be made with your oncologist.

Forms of BHRT: What Is Available

Let us walk through the various delivery methods and what each offers.

Estradiol Options

Transdermal Patches:

- Applied to skin (abdomen, buttocks, thigh)
- Changed 1-2 times weekly
- Deliver steady estradiol levels
- Bypass liver (lower clot risk than oral)
- Can sometimes cause skin irritation

Topical Gels and Creams:

- Applied daily to arms, thighs, or abdomen
- Absorbed through skin
- Flexible dosing
- Some women prefer this over patches
- Must wait for drying before contact with others

Oral Tablets:

- Convenient daily pill

- More convenient for some women
- Higher risk of blood clots than transdermal
- First-pass liver metabolism may be less ideal
- Generally, not my first choice unless transdermal is not tolerated

Vaginal Estradiol:

- Tablets, creams, or rings inserted vaginally
- Treats local symptoms (dryness, pain, urinary issues)
- Minimal systemic absorption
- Safe for most breast cancer survivors
- Can be used alone or with systemic hormones

Progesterone Options

Oral Micronized Progesterone:

- Capsules taken at bedtime
- Natural sedating effect aids sleep
- Protects uterine lining from estrogen
- Well-tolerated by most women
- Available as FDA-approved Prometrium or compounded

Topical Progesterone:

- Cream applied to skin
- Some women prefer this route
- Absorption can be variable
- May not adequately protect uterine lining in all women
- Often compounded

Vaginal Progesterone:

- Gel or suppositories
- Good absorption
- Can be used for uterine protection
- Sometimes preferred when oral causes sedation at inconvenient times

Important: If you have a uterus and take estrogen, you must also take progesterone to protect against endometrial hyperplasia and cancer. Estrogen stimulates uterine lining growth; progesterone keeps it in check.

If you have had a hysterectomy, progesterone is optional, but many women still benefit from it for mood, sleep, and breast health.

Testosterone Options

Topical Creams and Gels:

- Applied to vulvar area, inner thighs, or abdomen
- Often compounded since few FDA-approved options exist for women
- Improves libido, energy, muscle mass

Pellets:

- Implanted under skin every 3-6 months
- Steady hormone release
- Convenient (no daily application)
- Requires minor office procedure
- Cannot adjust dose once implanted

Dosing: Women need much smaller testosterone doses than men. Excessive testosterone can cause side effects like acne, hair growth, irritability, and adverse cholesterol changes. Careful dosing and monitoring are essential.

Dosing and Personalization

One of the most important aspects of BHRT is that **it is not one-size-fits-all.**

Starting low: Most providers start with lower doses and increase gradually based on symptom response. This minimizes side effects and allows your body to adjust.

Titration: Dose adjustments are common, especially in the first 3-6 months. What works initially may need tweaking as your body responds.

Route matters: Transdermal estrogen delivers different blood levels than oral. Compounded creams absorb differently than patches. Your provider considers both the dose and the delivery method.

Timing considerations: Some women need estrogen daily. Others do well with cycling patterns that mimic natural rhythms. Progesterone is often taken continuously if you have gone 12+ months without a period, or cyclically if you are still in perimenopause.

Monitoring: Regular follow-up is essential. Your provider will assess symptom relief, check for side effects, and sometimes order hormone level testing to ensure you are in the optimal range.

Safety Profile: What the Research Actually Shows

Let us address the fears head-on with current evidence.

Breast Cancer Risk:

The data is nuanced:

- Synthetic progestins (like those in Prempro) DO increase breast cancer risk
- Bioidentical progesterone does NOT appear to increase risk the same way
- Estrogen alone (in women without a uterus) shows minimal to no increased breast cancer risk in most studies
- The combination of bioidentical estradiol plus micronized progesterone has a more favorable risk profile than traditional HRT
- Risk is related to duration (longer use = slightly higher risk) and increases after about 5-7 years of use
- The absolute risk increase is small (around 1-2 additional cases per 1,000 women per year)

Cardiovascular Risk:

- Transdermal estradiol has lower cardiovascular risk than oral estrogen
- When started during perimenopause or within 10 years of menopause, estrogen may offer cardiovascular protection
- Bioidentical progesterone does not increase cardiovascular risk like synthetic progestins
- Women over 60 or more than 10 years past menopause may have increased risk; individualized assessment is essential

Blood Clot Risk:

- Transdermal estradiol has significantly lower blood clot risk than oral estrogen
- This is my primary reason for preferring patches or gels over pills
- Women with clotting disorders or history of DVT/PE are generally not candidates for systemic estrogen

Stroke Risk:

- Higher in women with certain risk factors (migraine with aura, hypertension, smoking)
- Lower with transdermal than oral estrogen
- Age matters: risk increases with starting hormones after age 60

The Bottom Line on Safety:

For healthy women starting BHRT in perimenopause or early menopause (before age 60 or within 10 years of final period), using transdermal estradiol with micronized progesterone, *the benefits typically outweigh the risks for symptom management and quality of life.*

The key is individualized assessment, appropriate screening, choosing the safest formulations, and regular monitoring.

What to Expect When Starting BHRT

First 2-4 weeks:

- Some women feel better almost immediately, especially with sleep improvement from progesterone
- Hot flashes may begin to decrease
- Breast tenderness is common initially (usually resolves)
- Mild bloating may occur as your body adjusts
- Vaginal bleeding or spotting can occur, especially if you are in perimenopause

4-12 weeks:

- Most symptoms continue improving
- Mood stabilizes
- Cognitive clarity improves
- Energy increases
- Vaginal symptoms begin resolving

3-6 months:

- Optimal benefits are typically achieved
- Side effects have usually resolved
- Dosing is dialed in
- You feel like yourself again

Ongoing:

- Regular follow-up every 6-12 months
- Dose adjustments as needed over time
- Annual breast exams and mammograms
- Monitoring for any concerning symptoms

Finding a Provider Who Prescribes BHRT

Not all doctors are comfortable prescribing bioidentical hormones. Some are not well-trained in menopause management. Others remain influenced by outdated fears from the 2002 WHI study.

Look for providers who:

- Specialize in menopause or bioidentical hormones
- Have completed training in hormone therapy
- Stay current with evolving research
- Listen to your symptoms and quality of life concerns
- Are willing to individualize treatment

Provider types who may prescribe BHRT:

- Gynecologists with menopause focus
- Functional or integrative medicine physicians
- Naturopathic doctors (in some regions)
- Nurse practitioners specializing in women's health
- Physicians specifically trained in bioidentical hormones

Telemedicine is increasingly available for menopause care, expanding access for women who do not have local providers experienced in BHRT.

The Decision Is Yours

I cannot tell you whether BHRT is right for you. That decision is deeply personal and depends on your symptoms, health history, risk factors, values, and goals.

What I can tell you is this:

BHRT is a safe, effective option for many women. When properly prescribed, using bioidentical hormones via optimal routes (transdermal estradiol, oral micronized progesterone), the benefits often dramatically outweigh the risks.

You deserve to feel good during this transition. If your symptoms are affecting your quality of life, you do not have to simply endure them. BHRT is one powerful tool in the integrative toolbox.

Fear should not be your primary decision-maker. Yes, hormones have risks. So does untreated menopause (bone loss, cardiovascular changes, quality of life impacts). The question is not whether hormones are risk-free (nothing is), but whether the benefits outweigh the risks for you.

In the next chapter, we will explore nutraceuticals—another powerful option that many women use alone or in combination with hormones. Understanding all your options empowers you to create the best plan for your unique needs.

ACTION STEPS

1. **Understand the difference between traditional HRT and bioidentical hormones.**
2. **Learn about both FDA-approved and compounded BHRT options.**
3. **Consider whether you are a good candidate** based on symptoms and health history.
4. **Review contraindications** and discuss with your healthcare provider.
5. **Research providers in your area** who are experienced in prescribing BHRT.
6. **Write down your questions** about hormones to discuss at your appointment.
7. **Remember: this is YOUR decision**, gather information, weigh options, and choose what feels right for you.

"I was terrified of hormones because of what I had heard. But when my doctor explained the difference between bioidentical and synthetic, showed me the current research, and discussed transdermal delivery, I felt confident trying them. Within a month, my hot flashes were gone, I was sleeping again, and I felt like myself for the first time in three years. I only wish I had started sooner."

Patricia, 52, Jamaica

CHAPTER 5

Nutraceuticals - Physician-Grade Supplements That Work

When I first started experiencing severe perimenopausal symptoms, I was hesitant about hormone therapy. Like many women, I wanted to explore other options first. I turned to supplements, but I quickly discovered that not all supplements are created equal.

The bottles at my local pharmacy contained underdosed ingredients, poor-quality extracts, and fillers that did nothing. I read the research and realized that the supplements proven effective in clinical studies used pharmaceutical-grade ingredients at therapeutic doses. not the watered-down versions sold in most stores.

That frustration led me to create the NoPause product line: physician-formulated nutraceuticals using the same quality ingredients and dosages proven effective in research. I focused on the two most disruptive symptoms women face, hot flashes, and mood changes, because I wanted to create solutions that would make the biggest difference in daily quality of life.

What Are Nutraceuticals?

The term "nutraceutical" combines "nutrition" and "pharmaceutical", it refers to supplements derived from food sources that provide health benefits beyond basic nutrition.

Unlike pharmaceuticals (synthetic drugs), nutraceuticals work with your body's natural processes. They provide nutrients, plant compounds, or other substances that support your body's ability to function optimally during hormonal transitions. **Nutraceuticals are not weaker alternatives to medications.** When properly formulated with high-quality ingredients at therapeutic doses, they can be remarkably effective, sometimes as effective as medications for certain symptoms, and often with fewer side effects. The key phrase is "properly formulated with high-quality ingredients at therapeutic doses." This is where most over-the-counter supplements fall short.

Why Quality Matters: Not All Supplements Are Equal

This is perhaps the most important section in this chapter. Understanding quality differences will save you money, frustration, and wasted time.

The Supplement Industry Problem

Unlike pharmaceuticals, dietary supplements are not tightly regulated. In many countries, including the United States, supplements do not require pre-market approval. Companies can sell products without proving they contain what the label claims or that they work.

Studies have shown alarming problems:

- Many supplements contain fewer active ingredients than claimed (sometimes none at all)
- Some contain contaminants (heavy metals, pesticides, unlisted ingredients)
- Quality and potency vary dramatically between brands
- The form of an ingredient matters (some forms are not well absorbed)
- Standardization is often absent (inconsistent amounts of active compounds)

This is why you can take one brand and feel nothing, then take a pharmaceutical-grade version and experience significant relief. The difference is quality, purity, standardization, and dose.

What "Pharmaceutical-Grade" or "Physician-Grade" Means

Pharmaceutical-grade or physician-grade supplements meet higher standards:

Purity: At least 99% pure with no binders, fillers, excipients, dyes, or unknown substances.

Quality sourcing: Ingredients are sourced from reputable suppliers with certificates of analysis proving identity and purity.

Standardization: Active compounds are standardized to specific percentages, ensuring consistent potency batch to batch.

Testing: Third-party testing verifies that what is on the label is actually in the bottle at the claimed dosage.

Bioavailability: Ingredients are in forms your body can actually absorb and use (not the cheapest forms that pass through unabsorbed).

Good Manufacturing Practices (GMP): Manufactured in facilities that follow strict quality control procedures.

Clinical dosing: Uses the same doses proven effective in research studies, not underdosed amounts.

This is the difference between supplements that work and supplements that are a waste of money.

The NoPause Product Line: Physician-Formulated Solutions

Now let me share why I created NoPause Hot Flashes Support and NoPause Mood Support, and what makes them different.

After experiencing my own perimenopausal crisis, nearly fainting in the operating room, I began researching every evidence-based solution. I tried numerous supplements, but most disappointed me. The doses were too low. The ingredients were not standardized. The formulations did not match what research showed worked.

I realized that if I wanted supplements that would help me and my patients, I needed to create them.

The NoPause Philosophy:

Every NoPause product is formulated based on three principles:

1. **Use only pharmaceutical-grade ingredients** at the doses proven effective in clinical research
2. **Combine synergistic ingredients** that work better together than alone
3. **Third-party test every batch** to ensure purity, potency, and safety

I do not cut corners. I do not underdose ingredients to save money. These products contain exactly what I would want for myself and my patients.

NoPause Hot Flashes Support

The Problem:

Hot flashes and night sweats are among the most disruptive menopausal symptoms. They interrupt sleep, cause embarrassment, drain energy, and make daily life miserable. While hormone therapy is highly effective, not every woman can or wants to take hormones. I wanted to create a natural alternative that actually worked, not just another underdosed supplement making empty promises.

What it contains:

This comprehensive formula combines seven evidence-based natural ingredients at therapeutic doses:

Sage Extract (Salvia officinalis): Sage has been used traditionally for centuries to reduce excessive sweating and hot flashes. Modern clinical studies confirm its effectiveness, one landmark study showed a 64% reduction in hot flash frequency after 8 weeks of use, with improvements seen across all severity categories. Sage appears to work by affecting sweat glands and thermoregulation centers in the brain, directly addressing the sweating component of hot flashes and night sweats. It modulates neurotransmitter activity and may have mild estrogenic effects. Sage is well-tolerated with minimal side effects, making it an excellent natural option for vasomotor symptoms.

Red Clover Extract (Trifolium pratense) - Isoflavones: Red clover contains naturally occurring isoflavones; plant compounds that have gentle estrogenic effects without being actual hormones. These phytoestrogens (biochanin A, formononetin, daidzein, and genistein) help fill the gap as your body's natural estrogen declines. Clinical studies and meta-analyses have shown that red clover can significantly reduce hot flash frequency, with many women experiencing substantial relief within 4-12 weeks of consistent use. Beyond hot flashes, red clover supports bone health by reducing bone loss, promotes cardiovascular function by improving arterial compliance and lipid profiles, and may improve skin elasticity and reduce aging signs. The isoflavones work gently and naturally, providing hormone-like benefits without the risks associated with synthetic hormones.

Ashwagandha Extract (Withania somniferous): This powerful adaptogenic herb helps your body respond more effectively to stress, which is crucial because stress is a major trigger for hot flashes. Ashwagandha has been extensively studied and shows remarkable benefits: it reduces cortisol levels by up to 30% in stressed individuals, significantly improves sleep quality and helps you fall asleep faster. Ashwagandha also supports balanced mood and reduces anxiety scores in clinical trials. It also enhances cognitive function, and reduces brain fog, increases energy and vitality, and improves overall resilience during hormonal transitions. Research consistently demonstrates that ashwagandha significantly reduces stress and anxiety while improving sleep quality, addressing multiple factors that worsen hot flashes. By calming the stress response and supporting restorative sleep, ashwagandha helps reduce both the frequency and intensity of vasomotor symptoms.

Fennel Seed Extract (Foeniculum vulgare): Fennel has a long history of use for women's hormonal health across many cultures. It contains phytoestrogens (primarily anethole) that provide gentle estrogenic activity, helping to balance hormone fluctuations during perimenopause and menopause. Clinical studies suggest fennel can reduce hot flash severity and frequency while also supporting digestive health and reducing bloating, which are common complaints during hormonal transitions. Fennel also has antioxidant and anti-inflammatory properties. Its mild estrogenic effects complement the other botanicals in the formula, contributing to overall symptom relief. Fennel is generally very well-tolerated and has been used safely for centuries.

Vitamin E (as d-alpha tocopherol): A powerful antioxidant that plays multiple roles in managing menopausal symptoms. Research shows that vitamin E at doses of 400-800 IU daily can reduce hot flash frequency and severity, one study showed a 50% reduction in hot flash scores. Beyond vasomotor symptoms, vitamin E supports cardiovascular health (critical as heart disease risk increases after menopause), protects against oxidative stress and cellular damage, promotes skin health, and reduces dryness, supports immune function, and may improve vaginal tissue health. Vitamin E appears to work by stabilizing vascular function, reducing oxidative stress, and potentially affecting hypothalamic thermoregulation. It is safe and well-tolerated at recommended doses.

Vitamin D3 (Cholecalciferol): Vitamin D deficiency is extremely common in menopausal women (over 50% are deficient) and can worsen symptoms while increasing health risks. Adequate vitamin D3 supports bone health and calcium absorption, which is critical for preventing osteoporosis as estrogen declines, mood regulation and reduces depression risk (vitamin D receptors are found throughout the brain), immune system function and reduces inflammation, muscle strength and reduces fall risk, cardiovascular health, and healthy blood pressure, and may reduce hot flash severity in deficient women. Vitamin D works synergistically with other ingredients in the formula, particularly with red clover for bone health and with the overall anti-inflammatory effects of the formula. Most women need supplementation to achieve optimal blood levels.

Folate (as Methylfolate/5-MTHF): The active form of folate (not folic acid, which requires conversion) is crucial for multiple body functions. Many women have genetic variations that impair folic acid conversion, making methylfolate essential. Folate supports mood regulation and neurotransmitter production (works with vitamin B12 to produce serotonin and dopamine), energy production at the cellular level, cardiovascular health by reducing homocysteine, healthy cell division and DNA synthesis, and cognitive function and memory. Folate deficiency is linked to depression, fatigue, and cognitive problems, these are all common during menopause. Including methylfolate ensures your body can immediately use this essential vitamin without needing to convert it, supporting mood, energy, and overall well-being during hormonal transitions.

Why this formula works:

Each ingredient addresses hot flashes and menopausal symptoms through different, complementary mechanisms. Sage directly reduces sweating and hot flash frequency through its effects on thermoregulation. Red clover and fennel provide gentle phytoestrogens that help balance declining estrogen levels. Ashwagandha reduces stress (a major hot flash trigger) and dramatically improves sleep quality. Vitamin E stabilizes vascular function and reduces oxidative stress. Vitamin D3 and folate support overall hormonal balance, bone health, mood, and well-being.

The combination creates a synergistic effect more powerful than any single ingredient alone. This multi-pronged approach addresses the complex physiology underlying hot flashes and night sweats, thermoregulation, hormone balance, stress response, vascular stability, and overall physiological resilience.

Expected results:

- Noticeable reduction in hot flash frequency and intensity within 2-4 weeks
- Maximum benefit by 8-12 weeks with consistent use
- Many women experience 50-80% improvement in vasomotor symptoms
- Night sweats often improve first (better sleep quality), followed by daytime hot flashes
- Better sleep quality as night sweats decrease
- Improved energy levels as sleep improves
- Reduced stress response and better emotional balance
- Overall sense of improved well-being

Who benefits most:

- Women with mild to moderate hot flashes who prefer not to take hormones
- Women who cannot take hormone therapy due to contraindications (breast cancer history, blood clot history, stroke history, liver disease)
- Women wanting to minimize hormone doses by adding natural support (can be used alongside low-dose BHRT)
- Women in perimenopause or post-menopause experiencing vasomotor symptoms
- Women seeking a pharmaceutical-grade natural solution backed by clinical research
- Women who want comprehensive support beyond just hot flash relief

How to use: Take as directed on the bottle (typically 2 capsules twice daily with food). Be consistent, benefits build over time with regular use. Allow 8-12 weeks for full effect, though many women notice improvement within 2-4 weeks. Do not stop taking it when you feel better, continue for sustained relief.

Safety: This formula is generally very well-tolerated. If you have a history of estrogen-sensitive cancers, discuss with your oncologist before using (due to red clover and fennel's weak phytoestrogen effects, though the risk is considered theoretical and low). Always inform your healthcare provider about all supplements you are taking, especially if you take any medications or have medical conditions.

NoPause Mood Support

The Problem:

The mood changes, anxiety, irritability, and depression triggered by hormonal fluctuations can be devastating. You feel like you are losing yourself. You cry over nothing. You snap at people you love. You lie awake with worry. You feel hopeless, empty, or overwhelmed.

Many doctors dismiss these symptoms ("just stress") or immediately prescribe antidepressants without addressing the hormonal root cause. I wanted to create a natural formula that supported the neurotransmitter systems most affected by declining hormones, providing real relief without the side effects of pharmaceutical antidepressants.

What it contains:

This comprehensive formula combines eleven evidence-based ingredients that support mood, reduce anxiety, improve sleep, and promote emotional balance:

Fenugreek Extract (Trigonella foenum-graecum): Fenugreek has been used traditionally to support women's hormonal health and has emerging clinical evidence for mood, metabolic, and hormonal benefits. It contains compounds that help balance blood sugar (which directly affects mood stability, blood sugar crashes trigger anxiety and irritability), support healthy hormone levels (may influence both estrogen and testosterone), reduce anxiety, and improve stress resilience, support healthy metabolism, and weight management, and has adaptogenic properties that help the body manage stress more effectively. Some research suggests fenugreek may support healthy testosterone levels in women (women need testosterone too, as it affects mood, energy, motivation, and libido). Fenugreek also has anti-inflammatory and antioxidant properties that support overall health during menopause.

Lemon Balm Extract (Melissa officinalis): This calming herb has been used for over 2,000 years to reduce anxiety, improve sleep, and enhance mood. Modern clinical research confirms that lemon balm significantly reduces anxiety and agitation, improves sleep quality without causing daytime drowsiness, enhances cognitive performance and reduces mental fatigue (particularly attention and memory), promotes a sense of calm and well-being, reduces stress-related symptoms, and has mild antidepressant properties. Lemon balm works by modulating GABA receptors (the brain's primary calming neurotransmitter system) and has acetylcholinesterase inhibitory activity that supports cognitive function. It is particularly effective for anxiety-related sleep problems and stress-induced mood changes. Studies show effects can be felt within hours, with greater benefits developing over weeks of use.

Milk Thistle Extract (Silybum marianum - Silymarin): While best known for liver support, milk thistle plays an important role in hormonal balance and mood during menopause. A healthy liver is essential for metabolizing and eliminating excess hormones, particularly estrogen. When liver function is optimal through milk thistle's hepatoprotective effects, hormonal balance improves, which directly affects mood, energy, and overall well-being. Milk thistle also has powerful antioxidant and anti-inflammatory properties that protect cells throughout the body, including brain cells. Additionally, some research suggests milk thistle may help reduce hot flashes in menopausal women by supporting healthy estrogen metabolism. It also supports healthy cholesterol levels and cardiovascular function.

Ashwagandha Extract (Withania somnifera): This powerful adaptogen appears in both NoPause formulas because of its comprehensive benefits for multiple body systems. For mood support specifically, ashwagandha reduces cortisol (the stress hormone) by up to 30% in clinical studies, significantly reduces anxiety scores—often as effectively as anti-anxiety medications, improves resilience to stress and promotes a sense of calm, supports healthy thyroid function (thyroid dysfunction often co-occurs with menopause and affects mood), enhances cognitive function including memory and processing speed, improves sleep quality and reduces insomnia, increases energy and reduces fatigue, and improves overall sense of well-being and quality of life. Research consistently demonstrates ashwagandha's effectiveness for reducing stress and anxiety while improving mood, which is essential for managing hormonally-driven emotional changes. Multiple high-quality studies support its use for anxiety and stress-related symptoms.

Saffron Extract (Crocus sativus): One of the most exciting natural mood-support ingredients with substantial clinical research backing. Multiple systematic reviews and meta-analyses show that saffron is as effective as some antidepressant medications (specifically SSRIs like fluoxetine and citalopram) for mild to moderate depression, significantly reduces anxiety and improves mood within 6-8 weeks, may improve sleep quality and reduce insomnia, has neuroprotective and antioxidant properties that protect brain health, and may reduce hot flashes and other menopausal symptoms. Saffron works by affecting serotonin, dopamine, glutamate, and other neurotransmitter systems. It also has anti-inflammatory effects and protects against oxidative stress in the brain. Saffron is well-tolerated and provides mood support without the sexual side effects, weight gain, or emotional blunting associated with pharmaceutical antidepressants. This is truly a remarkable natural antidepressant with solid research support.

L-Theanine: This amino acid from tea (particularly green tea) promotes calm alertness without sedation, a unique and valuable effect. L-Theanine increases GABA, serotonin, and dopamine (neurotransmitters essential for mood regulation and calm), induces alpha brain waves associated with relaxed focus and creativity, reduces stress and anxiety within 30-60 minutes of consumption, improves sleep quality without causing morning grogginess or dependence, enhances cognitive function, attention, and mental clarity, and reduces the negative effects of stress on the body. L-Theanine creates a sense of calm focus, reducing anxiety while maintaining mental clarity and alertness, which is perfect for managing the emotional volatility of hormonal transitions without sedation. It works beautifully with other mood-supporting ingredients in the formula.

Vitamin D3 (Cholecalciferol): Vitamin D deficiency is epidemic in menopausal women and strongly linked to depression, anxiety, and mood problems. Vitamin D receptors are found throughout the brain, particularly in areas that regulate mood and behavior. Adequate vitamin D3 supports serotonin production in the brain (the "feel good" neurotransmitter), significantly reduces depression risk and improves mood in deficient individuals, reduces inflammation throughout the body and brain (inflammation contributes to depression), supports healthy immune function, improves sleep quality and regulates circadian rhythms, supports bone and cardiovascular health, and works synergistically with B vitamins and magnesium for mood regulation. Vitamin D supplementation has been shown in clinical trials to improve mood, reduce depression risk, and enhance overall well-being during menopause. Most women need supplementation to achieve optimal blood levels (40-60 ng/mL).

Vitamin B3 (Niacin): Niacin is essential for energy production, brain function, and neurotransmitter synthesis. It supports conversion of food into usable cellular energy (critical for combating fatigue), healthy nervous system function and nerve signaling, synthesis of serotonin from tryptophan (one of the pathways for producing this mood-regulating neurotransmitter), reduction of inflammation throughout the body, cardiovascular health and healthy cholesterol levels, and skin health and repair. Adequate B3 is essential for maintaining energy, mental clarity, and stable mood during hormonal transitions. Deficiency causes fatigue, depression, brain fog, and irritability.

Vitamin B6 (Pyridoxine): Critical for neurotransmitter synthesis—your brain absolutely needs B6 to produce serotonin, dopamine, GABA, and other mood-regulating chemicals. Vitamin B6 supports mood regulation and significantly reduces depression risk, reduces severe PMS-like mood symptoms during perimenopause, supports cognitive function, and reduces brain fog, helps regulate sleep-wake cycles and supports melatonin production, works synergistically with other B vitamins, magnesium, and other nutrients, and supports immune function and reduces inflammation. B6 deficiency is common and worsens mood problems, anxiety, irritability, and sleep disturbances, making supplementation important during menopause. B6 is often called the "mood vitamin" because of its crucial role in neurotransmitter production.

Vitamin B12 (as Methylcobalamin): The active form of B12 that your body can use immediately without conversion. Many people have difficulty converting cyanocobalamin (the synthetic form) to active B12, so using methylcobalamin ensures optimal absorption and utilization. B12 supports nervous system health and nerve function, energy production and significantly reduces fatigue, mood regulation, and cognitive function (B12 deficiency causes depression and cognitive decline), red blood cell formation and oxygen delivery, cardiovascular health by reducing homocysteine, and healthy sleep-wake cycles. B12 deficiency causes profound fatigue, depression, brain fog, memory problems, irritability, and weakness; symptoms often mistaken for menopause alone or dismissed as "just getting older." Deficiency becomes more common with age as absorption decreases. Using methylcobalamin ensures you get the active form your brain and body need.

Magnesium Glycinate: The most absorbable, calming form of magnesium available. This essential mineral is involved in over 300 enzymatic reactions in the body and is absolutely crucial for mood, nervous system health, and sleep. Magnesium supports GABA function (the primary calming neurotransmitter that reduces anxiety), significantly reduces anxiety and promotes relaxation, improves sleep quality, duration, and helps you fall asleep faster, reduces muscle tension and physical manifestations of stress (tight jaw, tense shoulders, muscle aches), supports healthy blood pressure and cardiovascular function, helps regulate blood sugar levels (which affects mood stability), reduces inflammation, and is essential for activating vitamin D and producing energy. Magnesium deficiency is extremely common (over 50% of people are deficient) and worsens anxiety, irritability, insomnia, depression, muscle tension, and stress response. The glycinate form is gentle on the digestive system (does not cause loose stools like other forms), has superior absorption compared to oxide or citrate forms, and has additional calming properties from the glycine component. This is the gold standard form of magnesium for mood and sleep support.

Why this formula works:

Hormonal fluctuations during perimenopause and menopause deplete neurotransmitters, particularly serotonin (mood), GABA (calm), and dopamine (motivation and pleasure). Chronic stress elevates cortisol, which further disrupts mood, sleep, and hormonal balance. Poor sleep worsens mood. Blood sugar instability creates anxiety and irritability. It is all interconnected.

This formula works on multiple levels simultaneously to restore balance:

1. **Directly increases neurotransmitter production** (L-theanine, B6, B12, folate, niacin, magnesium)
2. **Enhances neurotransmitter function** (saffron, lemon balm)
3. **Reduces stress hormones** (ashwagandha, lemon balm)
4. **Supports hormonal metabolism and balance** (milk thistle, fenugreek)
5. **Provides essential cofactors** for all brain chemistry (B vitamins, magnesium, vitamin D)

6. **Reduces inflammation and oxidative stress** that damage mood-regulating brain areas (milk thistle, saffron, vitamin D, ashwagandha)
7. **Stabilizes blood sugar** to prevent mood crashes (fenugreek, magnesium)
8. **Improves sleep quality** (magnesium, lemon balm, ashwagandha, L-theanine)

This comprehensive, multi-targeted approach addresses the complex biochemical imbalances that hormonal changes create. You are not just masking symptoms, you are supporting your brain's ability to produce and properly use the neurotransmitters that regulate mood, sleep, stress response, and emotional stability.

Expected results:

- Improved mood stability and emotional balance within 2-4 weeks
- Reduced anxiety and greater sense of calm within 1-3 weeks (some ingredients like L-theanine work within hours, others take weeks)
- Less emotional volatility, tearfulness, and mood swings
- Reduced irritability, anger outbursts, and impatience
- Better stress resilience and ability to cope with challenges
- Improved sense of well-being, optimism, and life satisfaction
- Better sleep quality and easier time falling asleep (especially when anxiety interferes with sleep)
- Improved mental clarity, focus, and cognitive function
- More emotional stability throughout hormonal fluctuations
- Reduced frequency and severity of "meltdowns" or crying spells
- Greater patience and frustration tolerance

Who benefits most:

- Women experiencing hormonally-driven mood swings, anxiety, irritability, or mild to moderate depression
- Women who prefer not to take prescription antidepressants for hormonal mood changes

- Women wanting natural support alongside other treatments (can complement lifestyle changes, therapy, or low-dose hormones)
- Women in perimenopause with severe PMS-like emotional symptoms
- Women whose mood issues correlate with their menstrual cycle or hormonal changes
- Women experiencing anxiety that interferes with sleep
- Women who have tried antidepressants and experienced side effects or want a natural alternative
- Women dealing with stress-related mood problems during this transition

How to use: Take as directed on the bottle (typically divided doses throughout the day with meals for optimal absorption and sustained effect). Consistency is key, take it every day, not just when you feel bad. Benefits build over 2-6 weeks of consistent use, so commit to the full timeframe before assessing effectiveness. Some ingredients (like L-theanine) provide benefits within hours, while others (like saffron and ashwagandha) require several weeks for full effect.

Safety: This formula is generally well-tolerated with minimal side effects. Saffron can rarely cause mild digestive upset in sensitive individuals—taking it with food helps. The most important consideration: saffron, lemon balm, and other ingredients in this formula affect neurotransmitter systems. **Always check with your healthcare provider before starting this formula if you take any prescription medications,** especially:

- Antidepressants (SSRIs, SNRIs, MAOIs, tricyclics)
- Anti-anxiety medications (benzodiazepines)
- Sleep medications
- Blood thinners
- Diabetes medications (fenugreek may affects blood sugar)

While this formula can be an excellent alternative or complement to other treatments, discuss with your provider. Do not stop prescription medications without medical supervision.

Combining NoPause Products

Can you take both NoPause Hot Flashes Support and NoPause Mood Support together?

Absolutely yes. In fact, many women benefit from taking both products simultaneously, especially if they are experiencing both vasomotor symptoms and mood changes (which commonly occur together).

There are no contraindications to using both formulas together, the ingredients do not negatively interact. In fact, some ingredients provide overlapping benefits:

- Ashwagandha in both formulas supports stress reduction, sleep, and overall resilience.
- Vitamin D3 in both formulas supports bone health, mood, immune function, and overall well-being.
- Better sleep from reduced night sweats (Hot Flashes Support) improves mood.
- Better mood (Mood Support) may reduce stress-triggered hot flashes.

The combined approach:

- NoPause Hot Flashes Support addresses the physical discomfort of hot flashes and night sweats.
- NoPause Mood Support addresses the emotional and mental symptoms.
- Together, they provide comprehensive support for the two most disruptive symptom categories.

Many women find that addressing both areas simultaneously creates a synergistic improvement in overall quality of life, as feeling physically comfortable and emotionally balanced makes the entire menopausal transition more manageable.

Combining NoPause Products with Hormones

One of the most common questions I receive: "Can I take NoPause supplements if I am also taking hormones?"

The answer is yes. In fact, many women achieve optimal results using both.

The integrative approach:

Hormones address the root cause, replacing what your body no longer produces adequately. Nutraceuticals provide additional support, often allowing you to use lower hormone doses or addressing symptoms that hormones alone do not fully resolve.

Example combinations that work well:

For hot flashes:

- Low-dose estradiol patch (0.025-0.05 mg) plus NoPause Hot Flashes Support leads to excellent relief with minimal hormone dose. Some women can reduce their hormone dose when adding NoPause support.

For mood:

- Bioidentical hormones (estradiol + progesterone) for hormonal balance plus NoPause Mood Support leads to stable, positive mood and reduced anxiety. The combination often works great.

For comprehensive symptom relief:

- BHRT for hormonal foundation plus NoPause Hot Flashes Support plus NoPause Mood Support leads to multi-system support addressing physical and emotional symptoms

Many of my patients use this integrative approach and report better overall results than with any single treatment alone. The hormones stabilize the underlying hormonal chaos, while the nutraceuticals provide additional neurotransmitter support, stress adaptation, and physiological resilience.

Always inform your healthcare provider about all supplements you are taking. Most combinations are safe and beneficial, but monitoring ensures optimal results and safety.

When to Expect Results and How to Track Progress

Timeline for improvements:

Week 1-2:

- Some women feel benefits quickly (particularly from L-theanine in Mood Support, or reduced night sweats from Hot Flashes Support). Others may need more time, do not get discouraged.

Week 4-8:

- Hot flash reduction becomes noticeable (frequency and intensity decrease).
- Mood stabilization is more evident (fewer mood swings, less anxiety, better emotional control).
- Sleep quality continues improving as symptoms decrease.
- Energy levels improve.

Week 8-12:

- Maximum benefits typically achieved with consistent use.
- Hot flashes significantly reduced (50-80% improvement for many women).
- Mood is stable, positive, and resilient.
- Sleep is restorative.
- Overall sense of well-being is markedly improved.

Tracking your progress:

Keep a simple symptom journal to objectively measure improvement:

- Rate your top 3 symptoms daily (scale 1-10).
- Note sleep quality, mood, energy level.
- Track hot flash frequency (count them).
- Record any side effects or concerns
- Note overall sense of well-being

After 8-12 weeks of consistent use, review your journal. Are symptoms 30-50% better? That is meaningful, clinically significant improvement. Are you experiencing 60-70% improvement? That is excellent. No change at all? Consider whether you are taking the supplements consistently, whether the dose might need adjustment, or whether you need to add other treatments (like hormones).

Important: Nutraceuticals work with your body's natural processes, so they take time. Unlike medications that often work within days, natural supplements typically require 4-12 weeks for full benefits. Commit to at least 8-12 weeks of consistent use before deciding whether they are working. Do not stop too soon.

Global Availability and Access

NoPause products are available in:

- United States
- Canada
- United Kingdom
- Caribbean nations
- South Africa
- Online ordering with international shipping to many other countries

Visit www.nopausemd.com for current availability in your region and to order products.

For regions where NoPause products are not yet available, work with a healthcare provider to source pharmaceutical-grade versions of the key ingredients at therapeutic doses. The principles remain the same: quality matters, standardization matters, and clinical dosing matters. Use this chapter as a guide to understand which ingredients and doses are effective.

The Bottom Line on Nutraceuticals

High-quality nutraceuticals are not placebos. They are not "just vitamins." When properly formulated using pharmaceutical-grade ingredients at clinically effective doses, they are powerful therapeutic tools that can dramatically improve quality of life.

For some women, nutraceuticals like NoPause Hot Flashes Support and NoPause Mood Support provide sufficient relief on their own. For others, they work best in combination with hormones or other treatments. The key is using products that are formulated to work, not the underdosed, low-quality supplements that give the entire category a bad reputation.

I created NoPause Hot Flashes Support and NoPause Mood Support because I wanted solutions, I could trust for myself, for my patients, and for women everywhere who deserve better than what most supplement companies offer.

These formulas represent the best of what evidence-based natural medicine can provide for the two most disruptive aspects of the menopausal transition. They have transformed my life and the lives of countless women globally. They can help you too.

In the next chapter, we will discuss non-hormonal prescription medications, another tool in your integrative toolbox for women who cannot or prefer not to use hormones.

ACTION STEPS

1. **Evaluate whether hot flashes or mood changes are your most disruptive symptoms** to determine which NoPause product(s) to try.
2. **Consider trying NoPause Hot Flashes Support** if vasomotor symptoms are significantly affecting your quality of life.
3. **Consider trying NoPause Mood Support** if mood swings, anxiety, irritability, or depression related to hormonal changes are your primary concern.
4. **You can take both products together** if you are experiencing both hot flashes and mood changes.

5. **Give adequate time for results** (8-12 weeks minimum of consistent use) before deciding effectiveness.
6. **Track your symptoms** before starting and throughout treatment to measure improvement objectively.
7. **Discuss supplements with your healthcare provider**, especially if taking medications (particularly important for Mood Support due to potential interactions).
8. **Remember that pharmaceutical-grade quality matters more than price**, invest in supplements formulated to work synergistically with your body.
9. **Be consistent**, take the supplements every day, not just when symptoms are bad.
10. **Be patient**, natural supplements take time to build up in your system and create lasting change.

"I was skeptical about supplements after wasting money on brands that did nothing for me. But NoPause Hot Flashes Support actually worked. Within three weeks, my hot flashes decreased by about 60%. I could sleep through the night again. I added the Mood Support and my anxiety improved dramatically. These products gave me my life back. I tell every woman I know, quality matters."

Rebecca, 54, South Africa

CHAPTER 6

Non-Hormonal Medications - When You Cannot Take Hormones

Not every woman can take hormone therapy. Some have contraindications such as, breast cancer history, blood clotting disorders, active liver disease, or previous stroke. Others simply prefer not to take hormones for personal reasons. For years, women in these situations were told "just deal with it" or offered only minimal help. Thankfully, that has changed. We now have several FDA-approved non-hormonal prescription medications that effectively treat menopausal symptoms, particularly hot flashes. These medications are not as universally effective as hormone therapy, but for many women, they provide meaningful relief. In this chapter, we will explore what is available, how these medications work, who benefits most, and what to expect.

Understanding the Options

There are three main categories of non-hormonal prescription medications used for menopausal symptoms:

1. **Selective Serotonin Reuptake Inhibitors (SSRIs) and Serotonin-Norepinephrine Reuptake Inhibitors (SNRIs),** are antidepressants that also reduce hot flashes
2. **Gabapentin** is an anticonvulsant that reduces hot flashes and improves sleep
3. **Fezolinetant (Veozah)** is a newer medication specifically developed for menopausal hot flashes

Let us examine each category in detail.

SSRIs and SNRIs for Hot Flashes and Mood

These medications were originally developed to treat depression and anxiety, but researchers discovered they also reduce hot flashes, even in women who are not depressed.

How They Work

SSRIs and SNRIs affect neurotransmitter levels in the brain, particularly serotonin and norepinephrine. We believe they reduce hot flashes by:

- Stabilizing the hypothalamus (the brain's thermostat)
- Modulating serotonin receptors involved in temperature regulation
- Reducing the brain's sensitivity to fluctuating estrogen levels

For mood symptoms, these medications increase available serotonin and/or norepinephrine, which improves mood, reduces anxiety, and stabilizes emotions.

Specific Medications and Dosing

Paroxetine (Paxil):

- **FDA-approved specifically for hot flashes:** A low dose (7.5 mg) is FDA-approved under the brand name Brisdelle specifically for treating menopausal hot flashes
- **How effective:** Reduces hot flashes by 50-60% in most studies
- **Dose for hot flashes:** 7.5-10 mg daily
- **Dose for mood:** 10-40 mg daily (higher doses for depression/anxiety)
- **Timeline:** 1-4 weeks for hot flash reduction; 4-6 weeks for full mood benefits
- **Pros:** Only SSRI FDA-approved for hot flashes; effective for both vasomotor symptoms and mood
- **Cons:** Can cause weight gain, sexual side effects, and withdrawal symptoms if stopped abruptly

Venlafaxine (Effexor):

- **Type:** SNRI (affects both serotonin and norepinephrine)
- **How effective:** Reduces hot flashes by 50-60%, about the same as others but very effective
- **Dose for hot flashes:** 37.5-75 mg daily
- **Dose for mood:** 75-225 mg daily (higher for depression/anxiety)
- **Timeline:** 1-2 weeks for hot flash reduction; 4-6 weeks for mood benefits
- **Pros:** Very effective for hot flashes; also helps anxiety and depression; less weight gain than some SSRIs
- **Cons:** Can increase blood pressure at higher doses; withdrawal symptoms if stopped abruptly; may cause nausea initially

Escitalopram (Lexapro):

- **Type:** SSRI
- **How effective:** Reduces hot flashes by 40-50%
- **Dose for hot flashes:** 10-20 mg daily
- **Dose for mood:** 10-20 mg daily
- **Timeline:** 2-4 weeks for hot flash reduction; 4-6 weeks for mood benefits
- **Pros:** Well-tolerated; good for anxiety; effective for hot flashes and mood
- **Cons:** Sexual side effects; possible weight gain; withdrawal symptoms if stopped abruptly

Citalopram (Celexa):

- **Type:** SSRI
- **How effective:** Reduces hot flashes by 40-50%
- **Dose for hot flashes:** 10-20 mg daily
- **Dose for mood:** 20-40 mg daily
- **Timeline:** 2-4 weeks for hot flash reduction; 4-6 weeks for mood benefits
- **Pros:** Generally well-tolerated; less expensive (generic available)
- **Cons:** Sexual side effects; may prolong QT interval (heart rhythm) at higher doses

Fluoxetine (Prozac):

- **Type:** SSRI
- **How effective:** Reduces hot flashes by 40-50%
- **Dose for hot flashes:** 10-20 mg daily
- **Dose for mood:** 20-60 mg daily
- **Timeline:** 2-4 weeks for hot flash reduction; 4-6 weeks for mood benefits
- **Pros:** Long half-life means less withdrawal if you miss a dose
- **Cons:** Can be activating (increase anxiety initially); sexual side effects; not best choice for women needing tamoxifen (breast cancer treatment)

Desvenlafaxine (Pristiq):

- **Type:** SNRI
- **How effective:** Reduces hot flashes by 50-60%
- **Dose for hot flashes:** 50-100 mg daily
- **Dose for mood:** 50-100 mg daily
- **Timeline:** 1-2 weeks for hot flash reduction; 4-6 weeks for mood benefits
- **Pros:** Effective for both hot flashes and mood; once-daily dosing
- **Cons:** More expensive; can increase blood pressure; withdrawal symptoms

Who Benefits Most

SSRIs and SNRIs are particularly good choices for women who:

- Cannot take hormones (breast cancer survivors, history of blood clots)
- Experience both hot flashes and mood symptoms (depression, anxiety)
- Have a personal or family history of depression or anxiety
- Prefer to avoid hormones
- Need a medication that addresses multiple symptoms

Special consideration for breast cancer survivors: Women taking tamoxifen should avoid paroxetine and fluoxetine, as these can interfere with tamoxifen metabolism. Venlafaxine, desvenlafaxine, citalopram, and escitalopram are better choices.

Common Side Effects

Initial side effects (first 1-2 weeks):

- Nausea (taking with food helps)
- Headache
- Dizziness
- Increased anxiety or jitteriness (usually temporary)
- Fatigue or drowsiness (often improves)

Ongoing potential side effects:

- Sexual dysfunction (decreased libido, difficulty with arousal or orgasm), affects 30-50% of users
- Weight gain (varies by medication; paroxetine has highest risk)
- Dry mouth
- Constipation
- Sweating (paradoxically, even while treating hot flashes)

Withdrawal symptoms if stopped abruptly:

- Dizziness, vertigo
- Electric shock sensations
- Flu-like symptoms
- Mood changes
- Insomnia

Important: Always taper off these medications gradually under medical supervision. Never stop abruptly.

Realistic Expectations

SSRIs and SNRIs typically reduce hot flashes by 40-60%, which is meaningful but not complete elimination. Most women still experience some hot flashes, but they are less frequent and less severe.

These medications work best when combined with lifestyle strategies (cooling techniques, layered clothing, stress management) and possibly nutraceuticals.

For women with both hot flashes and mood symptoms, these medications can be particularly beneficial, as they address both issues with a single treatment.

Gabapentin for Hot Flashes and Sleep

Gabapentin is an anticonvulsant (anti-seizure medication) that has proven surprisingly effective for hot flashes, particularly nighttime hot flashes, and night sweats.

How It Works

The exact mechanism is not fully understood, but gabapentin appears to:

- Stabilize the hypothalamus (temperature control center)
- Reduce nerve excitability
- Improve sleep quality
- Potentially affect neurotransmitters involved in thermoregulation

Dosing and Use

Typical dose for hot flashes: 300 mg three times daily, or 300-600 mg at bedtime

Starting dose: Usually 300 mg at bedtime, then gradually increase as needed and tolerated

Maximum dose for hot flashes: 900-2,400 mg daily (divided doses)

Timeline: Hot flash reduction typically begins within 1-2 weeks

Effectiveness

Studies show gabapentin reduces hot flashes by approximately 45-55%, similar to low-dose SSRIs. It is particularly effective for nighttime hot flashes and night sweats. Many women find that taking the dose at bedtime addresses both night sweats and insomnia; a double benefit.

Who Benefits Most

Gabapentin is an excellent choice for women who:

- Cannot take hormones
- Experience primarily nighttime hot flashes and night sweats
- Have significant sleep disturbance
- Want to avoid antidepressants
- Have not responded well to SSRIs or SNRIs
- Have nerve pain or fibromyalgia (gabapentin treats these as well)

Side Effects

Common side effects:

- Drowsiness, sedation (this can be beneficial at bedtime but problematic during the day)
- Dizziness
- Fatigue
- Peripheral edema (swelling in feet and ankles)
- Weight gain (less common than with some SSRIs)
- Dry mouth

Important notes:

- Start with a low dose and increase gradually to minimize side effects
- Take the largest dose at bedtime if you experience daytime sedation
- Do not stop abruptly (taper gradually to avoid withdrawal)

- Use caution when driving or operating machinery until you know how it affects you
- Can be combined with SSRIs/SNRIs if needed

Realistic Expectations

Gabapentin works best for nighttime symptoms. Women who take it at bedtime often sleep better (from both reduced night sweats and the sedating effect). Daytime hot flashes may improve but often less dramatically than nighttime symptoms. The sedating effect can be either a benefit (helps sleep) or a drawback (daytime grogginess). Taking it only at bedtime maximizes benefit and minimizes daytime side effects.

Fezolinetant (Veozah) - The Newest Option

In 2023, the FDA approved fezolinetant (brand name Veozah), the first non-hormonal medication developed specifically and solely for treating menopausal hot flashes.

How It Works

Fezolinetant is a neurokinin 3 (NK3) receptor antagonist. This is an entirely different mechanism than hormones, SSRIs, or gabapentin. During menopause, declining estrogen causes increased activity in neurons that release neurokinin B. These neurons signal the hypothalamus that the body is overheating, triggering hot flashes. Fezolinetant blocks the NK3 receptors that respond to neurokinin B, essentially preventing the false "overheating" signal.

Dosing and Use

Dose: 45 mg once daily

Timeline: Hot flash reduction typically begins within 1-2 weeks, with maximum benefit by 4-12 weeks

Effectiveness

Clinical trials showed:

- Significant reduction in hot flash frequency (approximately 60% reduction)
- Significant reduction in hot flash severity
- Benefits maintained with continued use
- Some women experience near-complete resolution of hot flashes

Fezolinetant appears to be more effective than SSRIs or gabapentin for many women, approaching the efficacy of low-dose hormone therapy.

Who Benefits Most

Fezolinetant is an excellent option for women who:

- Cannot take hormones
- Experience moderate to severe hot flashes significantly affecting quality of life
- Have not responded adequately to SSRIs, SNRIs, or gabapentin
- Prefer a medication specifically designed for hot flashes (not an antidepressant or anticonvulsant)
- Want once-daily dosing
- Do not want the side effects associated with antidepressants

Side Effects

Clinical trials showed relatively few side effects:

Common side effects:

- Abdominal pain (usually mild)
- Diarrhea
- Insomnia (in some women)
- Back pain

- Hot flashes can temporarily worsen in the first few days (then improve)

Important monitoring:

- Liver function tests are required before starting and periodically during treatment
- Not recommended for women with liver disease or significantly elevated liver enzymes

Realistic Expectations

Fezolinetant appears to be highly effective for hot flashes in many women, as effective as low-dose hormone therapy. However, it only treats hot flashes. It does not help with mood, sleep (except through reducing night sweats), vaginal dryness, bone density, or other menopausal symptoms.

Cost consideration: As a new, brand-name medication, fezolinetant is expensive. Insurance coverage varies. This may be a barrier for some women despite its effectiveness.

Clonidine - An Older Option

Clonidine is a blood pressure medication that has been used off-label for hot flashes for decades, though it is less commonly prescribed now that we have better options. Must discuss thoroughly with your healthcare provider.

How It Works

Clonidine is an alpha-2 adrenergic agonist that reduces activity in the sympathetic nervous system (the "fight or flight" system involved in hot flashes).

Dosing and Effectiveness

Dose: 0.1-0.2 mg daily (oral tablets) or 0.1 mg weekly patch

Effectiveness: Modest—reduces hot flashes by approximately 20-40%

Who Might Consider It

Women who:

- Have high blood pressure (addresses both conditions)
- Have not responded to or cannot tolerate other options
- Need the least expensive option (generic available)

Side Effects

- Low blood pressure, dizziness
- Dry mouth
- Constipation
- Drowsiness
- Fatigue

Clonidine is generally not a first-line choice anymore since SSRIs, SNRIs, gabapentin, and fezolinetant are more effective with similar or better side effect profiles.

Oxybutynin - Off-Label Use

Oxybutynin is a medication approved for overactive bladder but has shown some benefit for hot flashes when used at low doses.

How It Works

Oxybutynin has anticholinergic effects that may influence sweating and thermoregulation.

Dosing and Effectiveness

Dose: 2.5-5 mg twice daily

Effectiveness: Studies show modest reduction in hot flashes, particularly reducing sweating

Side Effects

- Dry mouth (very common)
- Constipation
- Blurred vision
- Urinary retention
- Cognitive impairment (particularly concerning for older women)

Due to anticholinergic side effects and limited efficacy, oxybutynin is rarely used for hot flashes now that better options exist.

Choosing the Right Non-Hormonal Medication

With multiple options available, how do you decide?

Consider SSRIs or SNRIs if you:

- Have both hot flashes and mood symptoms (depression, anxiety, mood swings)
- Want one medication addressing multiple symptoms
- Are comfortable taking an antidepressant

Consider gabapentin if you:

- Experience primarily nighttime hot flashes and night sweats
- Have significant sleep problems
- Want to avoid antidepressants
- Have fibromyalgia or nerve pain (gabapentin treats these too)

Consider fezolinetant if you:

- Have moderate to severe hot flashes as your primary problem
- Have not responded adequately to other options
- Want a medication specifically designed for menopausal hot flashes
- Can afford it (or have insurance coverage)
- Do not have liver problems

Consider clonidine if you:

- Have high blood pressure
- Need an inexpensive option
- Have not responded to other medications

Work with your healthcare provider to choose based on:

- Your specific symptoms
- Your medical history
- Other medications you take
- Your preferences
- Cost and insurance coverage
- Side effect tolerance

Combining Non-Hormonal Medications

Sometimes, combining medications provides better relief than any single medication alone.

Common effective combinations:

Gabapentin at night + SSRI during the day:

- Gabapentin addresses night sweats and improves sleep
- SSRI addresses daytime hot flashes and mood
- Different mechanisms create synergistic effect

Fezolinetant Plus SSRI:

- Fezolinetant addresses hot flashes
- SSRI addresses mood symptoms
- No significant drug interactions

Important: Always discuss combinations with your healthcare provider. Some combinations are safe and effective; others may increase side effects or have interactions.

Combining Non-Hormonal Medications with Other Treatments

Non-hormonal medications plus nutraceuticals: This combination often works very well. For example:

- SSRI (for mood and hot flashes) plus NoPause Hot Flashes Support (additional hot flash relief)
- Gabapentin (for night sweats and sleep) plus NoPause Mood Support (for daytime mood)

Non-hormonal medications plus vaginal estrogen: Even if you cannot take systemic hormones, vaginal estrogen is often safe and can be combined with non-hormonal medications to address vaginal dryness and painful intercourse.

Non-hormonal medications plus lifestyle strategies: Always combine any medication approach with lifestyle optimization:

- Stress management
- Sleep hygiene
- Cooling strategies
- Regular exercise
- Healthy nutrition
- Weight management

The integrative approach, using multiple strategies that work through different mechanisms typically provides the best outcomes.

What These Medications Do Not Address

It is important to understand what non-hormonal medications do and do not treat:

What they treat:

- Hot flashes and night sweats (primary benefit)
- Mood symptoms (if using SSRIs/SNRIs)
- Sleep (particularly gabapentin)

What they do not treat:

- Vaginal dryness and atrophy (need vaginal estrogen or moisturizers)
- Bone density loss (need bone-building strategies)
- Cognitive symptoms (may help indirectly through improved sleep and mood)
- Weight gain and metabolic changes
- Skin changes
- Hair loss

Non-hormonal medications are targeted treatments for specific symptoms, primarily hot flashes. They are valuable tools but do not provide the comprehensive benefits that hormone therapy offers.

For symptoms they do not address, you will need additional strategies: vaginal moisturizers or estrogen, bone-building exercise and supplements, cognitive support strategies, metabolic management approaches, etc.

Making the Decision

If you cannot or prefer not to take hormone therapy, non-hormonal medications offer real relief, particularly for hot flashes and (with SSRIs/SNRIs) mood symptoms.

Questions to ask your healthcare provider:

1. Which non-hormonal medication do you recommend for my specific situation and why?
2. What results should I realistically expect?
3. How long until I notice benefits?
4. What are the most common side effects and how can I minimize them?
5. Can this medication be combined with nutraceuticals or other treatments I am using?
6. Are there any drug interactions with my current medications?
7. What is the plan if this medication does not work adequately?
8. How long might I need to take this medication?
9. What is the cost and is it covered by my insurance?

Remember:

- These medications are not as universally effective as hormone therapy, but they provide meaningful relief for many women
- You may need to try more than one medication to find what works best for you
- Combining medications (under medical supervision) may enhance results
- An integrative approach combining medication with lifestyle strategies and nutraceuticals often works best
- You deserve treatment. Please do not let anyone tell you to "just deal with" severe symptoms

In the next chapter, we will explore lifestyle medicine; the foundational strategies that support every other treatment and sometimes provide sufficient relief on their own.

ACTION STEPS

1. **Evaluate whether non-hormonal medications are appropriate for your situation** (contraindications to hormones, personal preference).
2. **Identify your primary symptoms** to help choose which medication might work best.
3. **Research costs and insurance coverage** for different options before deciding.
4. **Discuss options with your healthcare provider** using the questions provided above.
5. **Set realistic expectations**, these medications reduce symptoms but rarely eliminate them completely.
6. **Give adequate time** (4-8 weeks minimum) to assess effectiveness before switching.
7. **Consider an integrative approach** combining medication with nutraceuticals and lifestyle strategies.
8. **Track your symptoms** before and during treatment to objectively measure improvement.

"After my breast cancer diagnosis, hormones were not an option. My oncologist prescribed venlafaxine for my severe hot flashes, and within two weeks, they decreased by about 50%. Combined with

NoPause Hot Flashes Support and lifestyle changes, I went from 20 hot flashes per day to 3-4 manageable ones. I have my life back."

Carol, 56, United Kingdom

CHAPTER 7

Lifestyle Medicine - The Foundation That Changes Everything

When women come to my practice desperately seeking relief from perimenopausal or menopausal symptoms, they often want an immediate fix like a hormone prescription, a supplement, a medication that will make everything better. I understand that urgency. I felt it myself when I was suffering. But here is what I have learned both personally and professionally: **no treatment, not hormones, not supplements, not medications, will work optimally without the foundation of healthy lifestyle habits.** Lifestyle strategies amplify whatever other treatments you are using. Hormones work better. Supplements are more effective. Medications provide greater relief. Everything works synergistically when your lifestyle supports your physiology.

This chapter covers six foundational pillars of lifestyle medicine for perimenopause and menopause: nutrition, movement, sleep hygiene, stress management, gut health, and environmental toxin reduction. You do not need to be perfect in all six areas. Even small improvements create meaningful benefits. Let us explore each pillar and give you practical, actionable strategies you can implement immediately.

PILLAR 1: Nutrition - Food as Medicine

The foods you eat directly influence your hormones, inflammation levels, neurotransmitter production, and symptom severity. Nutrition is not about perfection or restriction; it is about making choices that support your body during this transition.

The Anti-Inflammatory Foundation

Hormonal changes increase inflammation throughout your body. Inflammation worsens virtually every menopausal symptom: hot flashes, joint pain, brain fog, mood changes, and long-term disease risk.

Anti-inflammatory eating emphasizes:

Vegetables (especially non-starchy vegetables): Aim for 5-7 servings daily. Focus on colorful options, leafy greens, cruciferous vegetables (broccoli, cauliflower, Brussels sprouts, cabbage), peppers, tomatoes, carrots. These provide antioxidants, fiber, and nutrients that reduce inflammation.

Fruits (particularly berries): 2-3 servings daily. Berries are especially beneficial, blueberries, strawberries, raspberries are packed with antioxidants that combat oxidative stress.

Healthy fats: Omega-3 fatty acids from fatty fish (salmon, sardines, mackerel), walnuts, flaxseeds, chia seeds. Olive oil, avocados, nuts. These fats reduce inflammation and support brain health, hormone production, and cardiovascular function.

Quality protein: Adequate protein is essential for maintaining muscle mass (which declines during menopause). Aim for 1.0-1.2 grams per kilogram of body weight daily. Include fish, poultry, eggs, legumes, Greek yogurt, cottage cheese.

Whole grains (in moderation): Choose minimally processed grains—quinoa, brown rice, oats, farro. These provide fiber and steady energy without blood sugar spikes.

Foods That Support Hormone Balance

Cruciferous vegetables: Broccoli, cauliflower, kale, Brussels sprouts, cabbage contain compounds (like indole-3-carbinol and DIM) that support healthy estrogen metabolism, helping your body process and eliminate estrogen safely.

Flaxseeds: Rich in lignans (phytoestrogens) that provide gentle estrogenic effects and fiber that supports elimination of excess hormones. Grind fresh and add 1-2 tablespoons to smoothies, yogurt, or oatmeal daily.

Soy (fermented forms): Tempeh, miso, natto contain isoflavones that can reduce hot flashes and provide mild estrogenic effects. Not all women benefit, but many do. Aim for 1-2 servings daily if tolerated.

Sesame seeds: Contain lignans that support hormone balance. Tahini (sesame seed paste) is an easy way to incorporate these. **Moringa** may also help alleviate hot flashes as it contains phytoestrogens-plant compounds that mimic the effects of estrogen on the body.

Foods That Stabilize Blood Sugar

Blood sugar fluctuations worsen hot flashes, mood swings, energy crashes, and weight gain. Stable blood sugar is crucial.

Strategies for blood sugar stability:

Combine protein with carbohydrates: Never eat carbs alone. Pair fruit with nuts, bread with eggs, oatmeal with Greek yogurt. Protein and fat slow carbohydrate absorption.

Prioritize protein at breakfast: Starting your day with adequate protein (20-30 grams) stabilizes blood sugar for hours and reduces cravings later.

Limit refined carbohydrates and sugar: White bread, pastries, candy, sugary drinks cause rapid blood sugar spikes followed by crashes. These spikes trigger insulin surges that worsen hot flashes and promote abdominal fat storage.

Eat regularly: Do not skip meals. Going too long without eating causes blood sugar drops that trigger stress hormones and worsen symptoms.

Consider the order of eating: Some research suggests eating vegetables and protein before carbohydrates reduce post-meal blood sugar spikes. This is called "carb sequencing."

Foods to Minimize or Avoid

Sugar and refined carbohydrates: These spike blood sugar, increase inflammation, worsen hot flashes, promote weight gain, and accelerate aging.

Alcohol: Triggers hot flashes, disrupts sleep, worsens mood, increases breast cancer risk, and adds empty calories. If you drink, limit to 3-4 drinks per week maximum, ideally less.

Caffeine: Can trigger hot flashes and worsen anxiety and insomnia in sensitive women. If you consume caffeine, avoid it after 2 PM and monitor whether it worsens symptoms. Some women tolerate it fine; others need to eliminate it.

Processed foods: Packaged snacks, fast food, processed meats contain inflammatory oils, excessive sodium, preservatives, and additives that increase inflammation and worsen symptoms.

Spicy foods: Trigger hot flashes in many women. Notice your response and adjust accordingly.

Practical Nutrition Strategies

The 80/20 approach: Eat nutrient-dense, anti-inflammatory foods 80% of the time. Allow flexibility 20% of the time. The Mediterranean diet is a great option for some women during the perimenopause and menopause journey.

Meal prep basics: Prepare vegetables, proteins, and whole grains in advance so healthy choices are convenient when you are tired or busy.

Hydration: Drink adequate water (aim for half your body weight in ounces daily). Dehydration worsens fatigue, brain fog, and dry skin.

Timing matters: Some women do better with three meals daily. Others benefit from smaller, more frequent meals that keep blood sugar stable. Experiment to find what works for your body.

Individualization: No single diet is perfect for everyone. Some women thrive on plant-based eating. Others need more animal protein. Pay attention to how foods make you feel and adjust accordingly.

PILLAR 2: Movement - Exercise for Hormone Health

Exercise is essential, particularly during perimenopause and menopause. It reduces hot flashes, improves mood and sleep, maintains muscle mass, protects bone density, supports healthy weight, and reduces disease risk. The key is finding the right type, intensity, and amount of exercise for this life stage.

Strength Training - The Non-Negotiable

If you do only one type of exercise during perimenopause and menopause, make it strength training.

Why it matters:

- Preserves and builds muscle mass (which declines 3-8% per decade after age 30, accelerating during menopause)
- Maintains metabolic rate (muscle burns more calories than fat, even at rest)
- Protects bone density (weight-bearing resistance exercise stimulates bone formation)
- Improves insulin sensitivity (reducing diabetes and weight gain risk)
- Enhances mood and cognitive function
- Increases strength and functional capacity for daily activities

How to do it:

- Aim for 2-4 sessions per week
- Target all major muscle groups (legs, back, chest, shoulders, arms, core)

- Use challenging weights (you should feel fatigued in the last 2-3 reps of each set)
- Focus on compound movements (squats, lunges, deadlifts, rows, presses)
- Work with a trainer initially if you are new to strength training

Options:

- Free weights (dumbbells, kettlebells)
- Resistance bands
- Weight machines
- Bodyweight exercises (push-ups, squats, planks)
- Classes (Body Pump, strength-focused group fitness)

Progressive overload: Gradually increase weight, reps, or intensity over time. Your muscles need ongoing challenge to adapt and grow.

Cardiovascular Exercise - For Heart and Mood

Cardio supports cardiovascular health, burns calories, improves mood through endorphin release, and reduces stress.

How much: 150-300 minutes per week of moderate-intensity activity, or 75-150 minutes of vigorous activity

What counts:

- Brisk walking
- Jogging or running
- Cycling
- Swimming
- Dancing
- Hiking
- Cardio classes (Zumba, step, kickboxing)
- Elliptical or rowing machine

Important balance: While cardio is beneficial, excessive cardio (especially without adequate strength training) can accelerate muscle loss and may not provide the metabolic benefits you need during menopause. Prioritize strength training, then add cardio.

Flexibility and Balance - Often Overlooked

Yoga: Combines flexibility, balance, strength, and stress reduction. Studies show yoga can reduce hot flashes, improve sleep, and decrease anxiety. Aim for 1-3 sessions weekly.

Stretching: Maintains range of motion, reduces injury risk, and feels good. Spend 5-10 minutes stretching after workouts or before bed.

Balance training: Becomes increasingly important as we age. Practice standing on one leg, use a balance board, or take tai chi classes. This reduces fall risk and maintains functional independence.

High-Intensity Interval Training (HIIT) - Proceed with Caution

HIIT involves short bursts of very intense exercise alternated with rest periods. It can be time-efficient and effective for fitness and fat loss.

However: During perimenopause and menopause, excessive high-intensity exercise can:

- Increase cortisol (stress hormone) when your body is already stressed
- Worsen sleep and anxiety in some women
- Increase injury risk
- Not provide enough stimulus for muscle building

If you do HIIT:

- Limit to 1-2 sessions per week maximum
- Ensure adequate recovery between sessions
- Do not do HIIT if you are already stressed, sleeping poorly, or experiencing high anxiety
- Consider lower-intensity steady-state cardio instead if HIIT worsens symptoms

Finding Your Exercise Sweet Spot

More is not always better. During hormonal transitions, your body needs:

- Adequate challenge to stimulate adaptation
- Adequate recovery to adapt
- Variety to address different needs (strength, cardio, flexibility)
- Consistency over perfection

Warning signs you are overdoing it:

- Worsening sleep
- Increased anxiety or mood problems
- Persistent fatigue
- Frequent injuries
- Not recovering between workouts
- Weight gain despite increased exercise

If you experience these, reduce intensity or volume and prioritize recovery.

Movement Throughout the Day

Formal exercise is crucial, but daily movement matters too:

- Take the stairs
- Park farther away
- Walk during phone calls
- Do squats while brushing teeth
- Stretch while watching television
- Garden, clean, play with children or pets

Non-exercise activity thermogenesis (NEAT), all the movement outside formal exercise, can significantly impact metabolic health and calorie expenditure.

PILLAR 3: Sleep Hygiene - Reclaiming Restorative Rest

Poor sleep worsens every menopausal symptom. Hot flashes increase. Mood deteriorates. Cognition suffers. Weight gain accelerates. Energy levels decrease. Sleep disturbance is one of the most common complaints during this transition. While hormones, supplements, or medications may be necessary to restore sleep, optimizing sleep hygiene is foundational.

Creating the Ideal Sleep Environment

Temperature: If possible, keep your bedroom cool (60-67°F or 15-19°C). Declining estrogen disrupts temperature regulation, but a cool room compensates. Use cooling sheets, moisture-wicking sleepwear, or a cooling mattress pad if needed.

Darkness: Your room should be completely dark. Light suppresses melatonin production. Use blackout curtains or an eye mask.

Noise: Minimize disruptive sounds. Use earplugs or a white noise machine if necessary.

Comfortable bedding: Invest in a supportive mattress and pillows. You spend one-third of your life in bed, this matters.

Remove screens: Avoid having, television, phone, or tablet in the bedroom. The bedroom is for sleep and intimacy.

Establishing a Consistent Sleep Schedule

If possible, go to bed and wake at the same time daily, even on weekends. Your body's circadian rhythm thrives on consistency.

Create a wind-down routine: 30-60 minutes before bed, engage in calming activities:

- Gentle stretching
- Reading (not on a screen)
- Taking a warm bath

- Meditation or deep breathing
- Journaling
- Listening to calming music

This signals your body that sleep is approaching.

Light Exposure Strategies

Morning light exposure: Get bright light (ideally sunlight) within 30-60 minutes of waking. This sets your circadian rhythm and supports nighttime melatonin production. Even 10-15 minutes helps.

Limit evening blue light: Blue light from screens suppresses melatonin. Avoid screens 1-2 hours before bed, or use blue light blocking glasses if you must use devices.

Dim lights in the evening: Lower indoor lighting 2-3 hours before bed. This naturally supports melatonin production.

Food and Beverage Timing

Avoid caffeine after early afternoon: Caffeine has a half-life of 5-6 hours. Even caffeine consumed at 3 PM can affect sleep at 10 PM.

Limit alcohol: While alcohol may help you fall asleep, it disrupts sleep architecture, causes middle-of-night awakenings, and worsens night sweats. Avoid alcohol within 3-4 hours of bedtime.

Do not eat large meals close to bedtime: Finish dinner 2-3 hours before sleep. Lying down with a full stomach can cause reflux and disrupt sleep.

A small protein-containing snack may help: Some women sleep better with a small snack before bed that includes protein and fat (Greek yogurt, nut butter on whole grain crackers). This prevents blood sugar drops that can wake you.

What to Do If You Cannot Sleep

Do not lie awake anxiously: If you cannot fall asleep within 20-30 minutes, get up. Go to another room, do something calming and non-stimulating (read a boring book, gentle stretching), then return to bed when sleepy.

Progressive muscle relaxation: Systematically tense and relax muscle groups from toes to head. This activates the parasympathetic (calming) nervous system.

4-7-8 breathing: Inhale for 4 counts, hold for 7, exhale for 8. Repeat 4-8 times. This triggers the relaxation response.

Avoid clock-watching: Turn the clock away from view. Checking the time increases anxiety about not sleeping.

When Sleep Hygiene Is Not Enough

If you are doing everything right but still not sleeping, you likely need additional interventions:

- Progesterone (if perimenopausal)
- Magnesium and other sleep-supporting supplements
- Sleep medications or nutraceuticals
- Treatment of underlying conditions (sleep apnea, restless legs syndrome)

Do not suffer in silence. Sleep is not optional; it is essential for health and optimum functioning.

PILLAR 4: Stress Management - Calming the Cortisol-Progesterone Connection

Chronic stress makes perimenopausal and menopausal symptoms significantly worse. Here is why:

Stress increases cortisol (your stress hormone). Elevated cortisol:

- Competes with progesterone production (your ovaries make both cortisol and progesterone from the same precursor, chronic stress shifts production toward cortisol)
- Worsens hot flashes
- Disrupts sleep (particularly causing 3-4 AM awakenings)
- Increases anxiety and mood problems
- Promotes abdominal fat storage
- Accelerates bone loss
- Impairs memory and cognition

Daily Stress-Reduction Practices

Deep breathing: Even 5 minutes daily makes a difference. Practice diaphragmatic breathing, slow, deep breaths into your belly. This activates your parasympathetic (calming) nervous system.

Simple technique: Breathe in for 4 counts, hold for 4, exhale for 6-8. The longer exhale triggers relaxation.

Meditation or mindfulness: Research shows 10-20 minutes daily reduces stress hormones, lowers blood pressure, improves mood, and reduces hot flashes.

Options:

- Guided meditation apps (Calm, Headspace, Insight Timer)
- Mindfulness meditation (focusing on breath, observing thoughts without judgment)
- Body scan meditation
- Loving-kindness meditation

Even 5 minutes is beneficial if you are new to meditation.

Journaling: Writing about stressors, emotions, or gratitude helps process stress and gain perspective. Morning pages (stream-of-consciousness writing first thing in the morning) clear mental clutter.

Nature exposure: Time in nature powerfully reduces stress. Walk in a park, hike, garden, or simply sit outside. Aim for 20-30 minutes daily if possible.

Connection: Social connection is a powerful stress buffer. Prioritize time with supportive friends and family. Join groups or communities that nourish you.

Creative activities: Art, music, crafts, cooking, or any creative pursuit engages your brain in ways that reduce stress and increase fulfillment.

Setting Boundaries

Perimenopause and menopause often coincide with demanding life stages—caring for aging parents, supporting teenagers or young adults, advancing careers. Many women are overwhelmed and overextended.

Learning to say no is essential:

- You cannot do everything
- Saying yes to everything means saying no to your health and well-being
- It is not selfish to prioritize your needs, it is necessary

Boundaries to consider:
- Limiting work hours or taking on fewer projects
- Delegating household tasks
- Saying no to commitments that drain you
- Protecting time for self-care
- Reducing exposure to toxic relationships or situations
- Your symptoms are telling your body it is stressed. Listen.

Professional Support

Therapy or counseling: If stress is overwhelming, anxiety is severe, or you are experiencing depression, professional support is crucial. Cognitive behavioral therapy (CBT) is particularly effective for menopausal symptoms.

Support groups: Connecting with other women navigating this transition reduces isolation and provides practical strategies.

PILLAR 5: Gut Health - The Gut-Brain Connection

Your gut microbiome, consists of trillions of bacteria living in your digestive tract, influencing hormones, mood, inflammation, immune function, and overall health.

Emerging research shows that gut health affects menopausal symptoms. Declining estrogen changes the gut microbiome, which can worsen symptoms. Supporting gut health improves outcomes.

Supporting Your Gut Microbiome

Eat diverse plant foods: The more variety in your diet, the more diverse your microbiome. Aim for 30+ different plant foods weekly (vegetables, fruits, legumes, nuts, seeds, whole grains, herbs, spices).

Include fermented foods: Yogurt, kefir, sauerkraut, kimchi, miso, tempeh, kombucha contain beneficial probiotics that support gut health. Include 1-2 servings daily.

Prioritize fiber: Fiber feeds beneficial gut bacteria. Aim for 25-35 grams daily from vegetables, fruits, legumes, whole grains, nuts, and seeds.

Consider a probiotic supplement: Quality probiotics can support gut health, particularly after antibiotic use or if you have digestive issues. Look for multi-strain formulas with at least 60 billion CFUs.

Minimize gut irritants:

- Excessive alcohol
- NSAIDs (ibuprofen, naproxen) when possible
- Unnecessary antibiotics
- Highly processed foods
- Artificial sweeteners (can disrupt microbiome)

Manage stress: Chronic stress damages gut health. The gut-brain connection is bidirectional, stress affects your gut, and gut health affects your mood and stress response.

Signs of Gut Dysbiosis

If you experience these, focus extra attention on gut health:

- Bloating, gas, irregular bowel movements
- Food sensitivities
- Skin issues (acne, eczema)
- Frequent infections
- Mood problems
- Brain fog
- Autoimmune conditions

Work with a functional medicine practitioner or gastroenterologist if gut issues are significant.

PILLAR 6: Environmental Toxin Reduction - Protecting Your Hormones

There are environmental chemicals, particularly endocrine-disrupting chemicals (EDCs), interfere with your hormones. During perimenopause and menopause, when your hormones are already in flux, reducing these toxic exposure, supports better outcomes.

What Are Endocrine Disruptors?

EDCs are chemicals that mimic, block, or interfere with your natural hormones. Common examples:

- **Xenoestrogens:** Chemicals that mimic estrogen (BPA, phthalates, parabens)
- **Heavy metals:** Mercury, lead, cadmium
- **Pesticides:** Glyphosate and others
- **Flame retardants:** PBDEs in furniture and electronics

These chemicals are everywhere around us; in plastics, personal care products, cleaning products, food packaging, water, and air. Complete avoidance is impossible, but you can reduce exposure significantly.

Practical Toxin Reduction Strategies

Reduce plastic exposure:

- Store food in glass, not plastic containers
- Never microwave food in plastic
- Avoid plastic water bottles (use stainless steel or glass)
- Choose fresh foods over canned when possible (can linings contain BPA)
- Avoid plastic-wrapped foods when possible

Choose cleaner personal care products:

- Read labels and avoid parabens, phthalates, triclosan, oxybenzone
- Use apps like EWG Skin Deep or Think Dirty to check product safety
- Choose fragrance-free products (fragrance often contains phthalates)
- Consider switching to cleaner makeup, shampoo, lotion, deodorant

Filter your water:

- Use a quality water filter (carbon filter or reverse osmosis) to remove contaminants
- Most tap water contains trace pharmaceuticals, pesticides, and heavy metals

Choose organic when possible:

- Prioritize organic for foods you eat most and foods on the "Dirty Dozen" list (strawberries, spinach, apples, grapes, etc.)
- Organic is ideal but expensive, do what you can afford
- Wash all produce thoroughly

Reduce household chemical exposure:

- Use natural cleaning products (vinegar, baking soda, castile soap)

- Avoid air fresheners and synthetic fragrances
- Open windows for ventilation
- Choose low-VOC paints and furnishings

Be mindful of receipts:

- Thermal paper receipts contain BPA, avoid handling them or decline receipts when possible

Eat lower on the food chain:

- Large predatory fish (tuna, swordfish) accumulate mercury. Do limit consumption
- Choose smaller fish (sardines, anchovies, salmon) lower in mercury

This is not about perfection. Make changes gradually. Even small reductions in toxic exposure support hormone health.

The 80/20 Rule for Lifestyle Medicine

If this chapter feels overwhelming, remember: you do not need to do everything perfectly to see benefits.

Aim for 80% adherence across all pillars. Make healthy choices most of the time, but allow flexibility. Rigidity and stress over perfection undermine the benefits of healthy habits.

Start with one or two changes that feel most doable. Once those become habits, add more.

Common starting points:

- Add strength training 2x per week
- Implement a consistent sleep schedule
- Practice 5-10 minutes of daily deep breathing or meditation
- Eliminate added sugar and reduce alcohol
- Switch to glass food storage containers

Small, consistent changes compound over time into transformative results.

When Lifestyle Medicine Is Not Enough

Lifestyle medicine is foundational and powerful, but it is not always sufficient on its own, particularly for moderate to severe symptoms.

You are not failing if you need additional treatment. Hormones, supplements, or medications are not signs of weakness. They are tools that, combined with healthy lifestyle habits, optimize your well-being. The goal is integrative care: lifestyle medicine as the foundation, with additional treatments layered on as needed for your unique situation.

Your Next Steps

You now understand the six pillars of lifestyle medicine for perimenopause and menopause. You have practical strategies for each area.

In the next section of this handbook (Part III), we will give you a 30-Day Jumpstart Plan that brings everything together, showing you exactly how to implement these strategies, track your progress, and create lasting change. But first, let me emphasize: **every positive change you make matters.** You do not need to overhaul your entire life overnight. Choose one or two strategies from this chapter that resonate with you. Start there. Build momentum. Your body will respond.

ACTION STEPS

1. **Review the six pillars** and identify which areas need most attention in your life.
2. **Choose 1-2 specific changes to implement this week** (do not try to change everything at once).
3. **Common high-impact starting points:**

   - Start strength training 2x per week
   - Eliminate added sugar and reduce alcohol

- Implement a consistent sleep schedule
- Practice 10 minutes daily of stress reduction
- Switch to glass food storage

4. **Track your changes and symptoms** to see what makes the biggest difference for you.
5. **Remember the 80/20 rule**, consistency matters more than perfection.
6. **Be patient**, lifestyle changes typically take 4-12 weeks to show full benefits.
7. **Celebrate progress**, every positive change supports your body during this transition.

"I thought I needed hormones to feel better. My doctor suggested trying lifestyle changes first; strength training, stress management, sleep hygiene, and cleaning up my diet. Within two months, my hot flashes decreased by 40%, I was sleeping better, and my mood was more stable. I eventually added NoPause Hot Flashes Support and got even better results. But those lifestyle changes were the foundation that made everything else work."

Jennifer, 48, Canada

PART III

YOUR PERSONALIZED ACTION PLAN

CHAPTER 8

Integrative Symptom Solutions - Quick Reference Guide

You have learned about hormones, nutraceuticals, medications, and lifestyle strategies. Now let us bring it all together with a practical guide for addressing specific symptoms using an integrative approach. This chapter is designed as a quick reference. Find your most troublesome symptom, see all your options at a glance, and understand how to layer treatments for optimal results.

Remember: start with lifestyle foundations, add targeted nutraceuticals or medications as needed, and consider hormones if symptoms are moderate to severe. This layered approach typically provides the best outcomes.

Hot Flashes and Night Sweats

Lifestyle Strategies (Layer 1 - Start Here):

- Keep bedroom temperature cool (60-67°F or 15-19°C)
- Use cooling sheets and moisture-wicking sleepwear
- Dress in layers you can easily remove
- Identify and avoid triggers (spicy foods, alcohol, caffeine, stress, hot beverages)
- Practice stress reduction (hot flashes worsen with stress)
- Maintain healthy weight (excess weight worsens hot flashes)
- Avoid smoking (worsens vasomotor symptoms)

Nutraceuticals (Layer 2):

- **NoPause Hot Flashes Support** (contains red clover, sage, fennel seed extract, ashwagandha, vitamin D3, folate and vitamin E at therapeutic doses)

- Individual supplements: Black cohosh (40-80 mg standardized extract), Pycnogenol (50-100 mg), Soy isoflavones (40-80 mg), Vitamin E (400-800 IU)
- Timeline: 4-12 weeks for maximum benefit

Non-Hormonal Medications (Layer 3):

- SSRIs/SNRIs: Paroxetine (7.5-10 mg), Venlafaxine (37.5-75 mg), Escitalopram (10-20 mg)
- Gabapentin (300-900 mg, particularly effective for nighttime symptoms)
- Fezolinetant/Veozah (45 mg daily, newest option specifically for hot flashes)
- Timeline: 1-4 weeks for benefit

Bioidentical Hormones (Layer 4 - Most Effective):

- Transdermal estradiol (patch or gel) - most effective treatment, 80-90% reduction
- Dose: Start low (0.025-0.05 mg patch or equivalent gel dose)
- Must add progesterone if you have a uterus
- Timeline: 2-4 weeks for maximum benefit

Integrative Layering Example:

- Start: Lifestyle changes plus cooling strategies
- Add: NoPause Hot Flashes Support
- If insufficient: Add low-dose transdermal estradiol plus progesterone
- Result: Comprehensive relief using multiple mechanisms

Sleep Disturbances

Sleep Hygiene (Layer 1 - Essential Foundation):

- Consistent sleep and wake times (even weekends)
- Cool, dark, quiet bedroom
- No screens 1-2 hours before bed
- Morning light exposure within 1 hour of waking
- Avoid caffeine after early afternoon

- Avoid alcohol within 3-4 hours of bedtime
- Relaxing bedtime routine (warm bath, reading, stretching, meditation)

Nutraceuticals (Layer 2):

- **NoPause Mood Support** (contains, lemon balm, milk thistle, saffron extract, ashwagandha, L-theanine, fenugreek extract, magnesium glycinate, vitamin B3, B6, B12 and vitamin D3)
- **Magnesium glycinate** (300-400 mg before bed) - supports GABA and melatonin
- **L-theanine** (200-400 mg before bed) - promotes relaxation without sedation
- **Melatonin** (0.5-3 mg, 30-60 minutes before bed) - regulates sleep-wake cycle
- Combination formula with valerian root, passionflower, 5-HTP
- Timeline: 1-2 weeks for noticeable improvement

Medications (Layer 3):

- **Gabapentin** (300-600 mg at bedtime) - particularly effective for sleep disrupted by night sweats
- **Low-dose trazodone** (25-50 mg) - sedating antidepressant
- **Prescription sleep aids** (used cautiously and short-term)

Bioidentical Hormones (Layer 4):

- **Progesterone** (oral micronized, 100-200 mg at bedtime) - natural sedating effect, supports deep sleep
- Estradiol (reduces night sweats that fragment sleep)
- Timeline: Progesterone often improves sleep within days to weeks

Integrative Layering Example:

- Start: Sleep hygiene plus address night sweats
- Start NoPause Mood Support
- If insufficient: Add oral progesterone at bedtime
- Result: Deep, restorative sleep through multiple mechanisms

Mood Changes, Anxiety, and Depression

Lifestyle Strategies (Layer 1):

- Regular exercise (particularly strength training and yoga)
- Daily stress management (meditation, deep breathing, journaling)
- Adequate sleep (mood deteriorates with poor sleep)
- Blood sugar stability (fluctuations worsen mood)
- Social connection and support
- Limit alcohol (worsens depression and anxiety)
- Morning light exposure (supports mood)

Nutraceuticals (Layer 2):

- **NoPause Mood Support** (contains, lemon balm, milk thistle, saffron extract, ashwagandha, L-theanine, fenugreek extract, magnesium glycinate, vitamin D3, and B vitamins at therapeutic doses)
- Individual supplements: St. John's Wort (900 mg standardized), 5-HTP (50-300 mg), L-theanine (200-400 mg), Magnesium Glycinate (300-400 mg), B-complex vitamins, Omega-3 fatty acids (1,000-2,000 mg EPA/DHA)
- Timeline: 2-6 weeks for mood stabilization

Medications (Layer 3):

- **SSRIs/SNRIs** if hormonal mood changes are severe: Escitalopram, sertraline, venlafaxine, desvenlafaxine
- These address both mood and hot flashes
- Timeline: 4-6 weeks for full mood benefits

Bioidentical Hormones (Layer 4):

- **Estradiol** (supports serotonin production, stabilizes mood)
- **Progesterone** (supports GABA, reduces anxiety)
- Combination often provides dramatic mood improvement
- Timeline: 2-4 weeks for noticeable mood changes

Professional Support:

- Therapy/counseling (CBT particularly effective)
- If depression is severe or includes suicidal thoughts, seek immediate professional help

Integrative Layering Example:

- Start: Daily stress management, plus exercise plus sleep optimization
- Add: NoPause Mood Support plus Omega-3s
- If insufficient: Add bioidentical estradiol plus progesterone
- Result: Stable, positive mood through neurotransmitter and hormone support

Brain Fog and Memory Problems

Lifestyle Strategies (Layer 1):

- Prioritize sleep (cognitive function deteriorates with poor sleep)
- Regular exercise (increases blood flow to brain)
- Mental stimulation (learning new skills, puzzles, reading)
- Stress management (chronic stress impairs cognition)
- Blood sugar stability (fluctuations worsen brain fog)
- Adequate hydration
- Limit alcohol

Nutraceuticals (Layer 2):

- NoPause Mood Support (supports brain function and memory)
- **Omega-3 fatty acids** (1,000-2,000 mg EPA/DHA daily) - essential for brain structure and function
- **B vitamins** (B6, B12, folate in active forms) - support neurotransmitter production
- **Ginkgo biloba** (120-240 mg standardized extract) - increases cerebral blood flow
- **Bacopa monnieri** (300 mg standardized) - enhances memory and processing

- **Phosphatidylserine** (100-300 mg) - supports brain cell membranes
- Timeline: 4-12 weeks for cognitive improvements

Bioidentical Hormones (Layer 3):

- **Estradiol** - crucial for brain metabolism, neurotransmitter function, memory
- Many women report dramatic cognitive improvement on estradiol
- Timeline: 4-8 weeks for cognitive clarity

Address Contributing Factors:

- Rule out thyroid dysfunction, vitamin B12 deficiency, sleep apnea
- Evaluate medications that impair cognition (antihistamines, sleeping pills, pain medications)

Integrative Layering Example:

- Start: Sleep optimization plus daily exercise, plus stress management
- NoPause Mood Support
- Add: Omega-3s
- If insufficient: Add transdermal estradiol
- Result: Mental clarity and sharp memory through multiple pathways

Weight Gain and Metabolic Changes

Lifestyle Strategies (Layer 1 - Most Important):

- **Strength training 2-4x per week** (maintains muscle mass and metabolic rate)
- Adequate protein intake (1.0-1.2 g per kg body weight daily)
- Blood sugar stability (protein with every meal, limit refined carbs and sugar)
- Stress management (cortisol promotes abdominal fat storage)

- Adequate sleep (sleep deprivation worsens weight gain and insulin resistance)
- Reduce or eliminate alcohol (empty calories, disrupts metabolism)
- Consider intermittent fasting if appropriate

Nutraceuticals (Layer 2):

- **Berberine** (500 mg, 2-3x daily with meals) - improves insulin sensitivity
- **Green tea extract** (400-500 mg EGCG daily) - modest metabolic boost
- **Chromium** (200-400 mcg daily) - supports insulin function
- **Alpha-lipoic acid** (300-600 mg daily) - improves glucose metabolism
- **Omega-3 fatty acids** (reduce inflammation, support metabolism)
- Timeline: 8-12 weeks for metabolic improvements

Bioidentical Hormones (Layer 3):

- **Estradiol** - improves insulin sensitivity, supports healthier body composition
- **Testosterone** (if deficient) - preserves muscle mass, supports fat loss
- **Progesterone** - balances estrogen, reduces bloating
- Hormones alone will not cause weight loss, but they support metabolic function

Medical Evaluation:

- Rule out hypothyroidism (very common in this age group)
- Check fasting insulin, glucose, hemoglobin A1c
- Evaluate for metabolic syndrome or prediabetes

Integrative Layering Example:

- Start: Strength training plus protein at every meal, plus eliminate added sugar
- Add: Berberine plus Omega-3s, plus stress management

- If needed: Add bioidentical hormones (especially if testosterone is low)
- Result: Improved body composition and metabolic health

Low Libido and Sexual Dysfunction

Lifestyle Strategies (Layer 1):

- Prioritize sleep (fatigue kills libido)
- Manage stress (chronic stress suppresses desire)
- Regular exercise (increases energy and body confidence)
- Communicate openly with partner
- Address relationship issues if present
- Reduce alcohol (impairs sexual response)

Address Vaginal Dryness First:

- **Vaginal estradiol** (cream, tablet, or ring) - restores vaginal tissue health
- **Vaginal Hyaluronic Acid cream**
- Water-based lubricants for immediate relief
- Regular sexual activity maintains vaginal elasticity

Nutraceuticals (Layer 2):

- **Maca root** (1,500-3,000 mg daily) - may increase desire
- **DHEA** (10-50 mg daily, requires medical supervision) - converts to sex hormones
- **L-arginine** (3,000-5,000 mg daily) - improves genital blood flow
- Timeline: 4-8 weeks for libido changes

Bioidentical Hormones (Layer 3 - Most Effective):

- **Testosterone** (cream or gel applied to vulvar area or inner thighs) - primary hormone for libido
- Dosing: Women need much smaller doses than men; start low
- **Estradiol** (systemic) - supports arousal and vaginal health
- **Vaginal estradiol** - essential for treating painful intercourse from vaginal atrophy

- Timeline: 6-12 weeks for libido improvement with testosterone

Important Considerations:

- Pain during intercourse must be addressed first (cannot desire something that hurts)
- Depression and anxiety medications (SSRIs) often reduce libido. Please discuss with provider
- Rule out other causes: hypothyroidism, prolactin excess, medications

Integrative Layering Example:

- Start: Address vaginal dryness with vaginal estradiol plus lubricants
- Add: Improve sleep plus reduce stress, plus communicate with partner
- If insufficient: Add testosterone (if deficient) plus Maca root
- Result: Restored desire and comfortable, pleasurable intimacy

Vaginal Dryness and Painful Intercourse

First-Line Treatment (Essential):

- **Vaginal estradiol** (Vagifem tablets 10 mcg, or creams 0.5-1 g, or ring)
- Used locally, minimal systemic absorption
- Safe for most women, including many breast cancer survivors (discuss with oncologist)
- Timeline: 2-4 weeks for noticeable improvement, 3 months for maximum benefit
- Must use regularly and long-term (symptoms return if stopped)

Vaginal Moisturizers:

- **Hyaluronic acid vaginal moisturizers** (use 2-3x per week)
- Different from lubricants (moisturizers provide ongoing hydration, lubricants for intercourse)

Lubricants for Intercourse:

- Water-based or silicone-based lubricants
- Avoid products with glycerin, parabens, or fragrances
- Use generously

Lifestyle:

- Regular sexual activity (maintains vaginal elasticity and blood flow)
- Adequate hydration
- Omega-3 fatty acids support tissue health
- Vitamin E suppositories may provide modest benefit

Systemic Hormones:

- Systemic estradiol (oral, patch, gel) helps but not as effective as local vaginal estradiol
- DHEA vaginal suppositories (Intrarosa/Prasterone) - FDA-approved for vaginal atrophy

Important:

- Do not suffer in silence - vaginal atrophy worsens without treatment
- Vaginal estradiol is remarkably safe and effective
- Pain-free intimacy is possible with proper treatment

Integrative Approach:

- Start: Vaginal estradiol (essential) + vaginal moisturizer
- Add: Water-based lubricant for intercourse + Omega-3s
- If insufficient: Add systemic estradiol or DHEA suppositories
- Result: Comfortable, pain-free intimacy

Bone Health and Osteoporosis Prevention

Lifestyle Strategies (Layer 1 - Essential):

- **Weight-bearing exercise** (walking, jogging, dancing) 3-5x per week
- **Strength training** (resistance exercise) 2-4x per week - critical for bone density
- Adequate protein intake (supports bone matrix)
- Do not smoke (accelerates bone loss)
- Limit alcohol (excessive alcohol weakens bones)
- Maintain healthy body weight (too thin increases fracture risk)

Nutrition (Layer 2):

- **Calcium** (1,000-1,200 mg daily from food and supplements combined)
- Best food sources: Dairy, leafy greens, sardines with bones, fortified foods
- Supplement if needed (in divided doses for better absorption)
- **Vitamin D3** (2,000-5,000 IU daily; aim for blood level 40-60 ng/mL)
- **Vitamin K2 (MK-7)** (90-180 mcg daily) - directs calcium into bones
- **Magnesium** (300-400 mg daily) - required for bone formation

Bioidentical Hormones (Layer 3 - Highly Effective):

- **Estradiol** - one of the most effective treatments for preventing bone loss
- Inhibits bone breakdown, supports bone formation
- Most beneficial when started in perimenopause or early menopause
- **Testosterone** (if deficient) - also supports bone density

Medications (Layer 4 - If Osteoporosis Present):

- Bisphosphonates (alendronate, risedronate)
- Denosumab (Prolia)
- Discuss with provider if DEXA scan shows osteoporosis

Testing:

- Baseline DEXA scan at menopause or age 65 (earlier if risk factors)
- Repeat every 1-2 years if concerning

Integrative Approach:

- Start: Weight-bearing exercise + strength training
- Add: Calcium + Vitamin D3 plus K2, plus Magnesium
- Add: Estradiol (if using hormones for other symptoms - bone protection is a bonus)
- If osteoporosis develops: Add bone-building medications
- Result: Strong, healthy bones for life

Joint Pain and Muscle Aches

Lifestyle Strategies (Layer 1):

- Regular movement (prevents stiffness)
- Gentle stretching and yoga
- Strength training (supports joints through muscle support)
- Maintain healthy weight (reduces joint stress)
- Apply heat or cold as needed
- Adequate sleep (pain perception worsens with poor sleep)

Nutrition (Layer 2):

- **Anti-inflammatory diet** (vegetables, fruits, omega-3s, minimal processed foods)
- **Omega-3 fatty acids** (2,000 mg EPA/DHA daily) - reduces inflammation
- **Turmeric/Curcumin** (500-1,000 mg with black pepper for absorption)
- **Ginger** (500-1,000 mg) - anti-inflammatory
- Eliminate inflammatory foods if sensitive (gluten, dairy, sugar)

Bioidentical Hormones (Layer 3):

- **Estradiol** - has anti-inflammatory properties; many women report significant joint pain reduction on estradiol
- Timeline: 4-8 weeks for pain improvement

Topical Treatments:

- Topical NSAIDs (diclofenac gel)
- CBD (cannabidiol) creams
- Arnica gel

Medical Evaluation:

- Rule out inflammatory conditions (rheumatoid arthritis, autoimmune conditions)
- Rule out vitamin D deficiency (causes muscle aches)
- Physical therapy if needed

Integrative Approach:

- Start: Anti-inflammatory diet plus regular movement plus Omega-3s
- Add: Turmeric plus stretching/yoga
- If insufficient: Add transdermal estradiol
- Result: Reduced inflammation and pain

Cardiovascular Health

Lifestyle Strategies (Layer 1 - Most Important):

- Regular aerobic exercise (150-300 minutes per week moderate intensity)
- Strength training (supports metabolic health)
- Anti-inflammatory Mediterranean-style diet
- Maintain healthy weight
- Do not smoke
- Limit alcohol
- Manage stress (reduces blood pressure and inflammation)
- Adequate sleep

Nutrition (Layer 2):

- **Omega-3 fatty acids** (1,000-2,000 mg EPA/DHA daily) - supports heart health
- Fiber (25-35 g daily) - lowers cholesterol
- Minimize trans fats, processed foods, excess sodium
- Healthy fats-olive oil and avocado oil.
- Increase vegetables, fruits, whole grains, legumes

Bioidentical Hormones (Layer 3):

- **Estradiol** (when started in perimenopause or within 10 years of menopause) - supports vascular health, improves cholesterol profiles
- Timing is critical - cardiovascular benefit is time-sensitive
- Use transdermal estradiol (lower cardiovascular risk than oral)

Medical Management:

- Monitor blood pressure, cholesterol, blood sugar regularly
- Treat hypertension, high cholesterol, or diabetes if present
- Consider aspirin if appropriate (discuss with provider)
- Know your cardiovascular risk factors

Integrative Approach:

- Start: Regular exercise plus anti-inflammatory diet, plus stress management
- Add: Omega-3s plus fiber-rich foods
- Add: Transdermal estradiol (if starting in perimenopause or early menopause)
- Medical treatment if needed for blood pressure, cholesterol, or blood sugar
- Result: Optimal cardiovascular health and reduced disease risk

The Layered Approach: Key Principles

1. **Start with lifestyle foundations** - these support every other treatment

2. **Add targeted nutraceuticals** - quality matters; use therapeutic doses
3. **Consider non-hormonal medications** if you cannot or prefer not to use hormones
4. **Add bioidentical hormones** if symptoms are moderate to severe and you have no contraindications
5. **Track your progress** - what gets measured gets improved
6. **Be patient** - most treatments take 4-12 weeks for full benefits
7. **Adjust as needed** - your needs may change over time
8. **Work with knowledgeable providers** - integrative care requires collaboration

This quick reference guide gives you a roadmap for the major symptom. In the next chapter, we will provide a step-by-step 30-Day Jumpstart Plan that helps you implement these strategies systematically and track your progress.

"This symptom-by-symptom guide changed everything for me. I could see all my options in one place and create a personalized plan. I started with lifestyle changes and NoPause products for my worst symptoms, then added hormones when I was ready. Within three months, I felt like myself again."

Rose, 51, United States

CHAPTER 9

The NoPause 30-Day Jumpstart Plan

Knowledge is power, but action creates transformation.

You have learned about hormones, symptoms, treatment options, and lifestyle strategies. Now it is time to put it all together into a practical, step-by-step plan you can start today.

This 30-Day Jumpstart Plan will help you:

- Identify your priority symptoms
- Implement foundational lifestyle changes
- Start targeted treatments
- Track your progress
- Build momentum toward lasting relief

The plan is designed to be manageable, adding new strategies gradually rather than overwhelming you with everything at once. Each week builds on the previous week, creating sustainable habits that support your well-being.

Let us begin.

Before You Start: Your Baseline Assessment

Before making any changes, take stock of where you are. This baseline helps you measure progress objectively.

Symptom Inventory

Rate each symptom on a scale of 0-10 (0 = not present, 10 = severe, life-disrupting):

Vasomotor Symptoms:

- Hot flashes (daytime): ___
- Night sweats: ___
- Frequency of hot flashes per day: ___

Sleep:

- Difficulty falling asleep: ___
- Difficulty staying asleep: ___
- Sleep quality overall: ___
- Feeling rested upon waking: ___

Mood and Mental Health:

- Depression or sadness: ___
- Anxiety or worry: ___
- Irritability: ___
- Mood swings: ___

Cognitive Function:

- Brain fog: ___
- Memory problems: ___
- Difficulty concentrating: ___

Physical Symptoms:

- Fatigue: ___
- Joint or muscle pain: ___
- Headaches: ___
- Weight concerns: ___

Sexual Health:

- Libido (desire): ___
- Vaginal dryness: ___
- Painful intercourse: ___

Overall Quality of Life:

- How much are symptoms affecting your daily life? ___
- How would you rate your overall well-being? ___

Identify Your Top 3 Priority Symptoms

Look at your ratings above. Which 3 symptoms are most disruptive to your quality of life? Write them here:

1.
2.
3.

These become your initial focus. You will address other symptoms too, but prioritizing helps you stay focused and motivated.

Current Habits Assessment

Rate your current habits (1 = poor, 5 = excellent):

- Nutrition quality: ___
- Exercise frequency: ___
- Sleep hygiene: ___
- Stress management: ___
- Alcohol consumption: ___ (frequency per week)
- Caffeine consumption: ___ (servings per day)

This shows which lifestyle areas need most attention.

Week 1: Foundation and Assessment

Your Week 1 Goals

This week focuses on establishing baseline habits and gathering information, not making dramatic changes yet. You are setting the foundation for success.

Goal 1: Track Everything

For 7 days, track:

- All symptoms (use the rating scale above, note severity and timing)
- Sleep (time to bed, wake time, quality, number of awakenings)
- Food and beverages (what you eat and drink, when)
- Exercise (type, duration)
- Stress levels (rate 1-10 at end of each day)
- Hot flash frequency and severity (if applicable)

Why: You cannot improve what you do not measure. This week gives you data to identify patterns. Maybe hot flashes correlate with certain foods, or mood crashes happen on days you skip exercise, or sleep is worst after alcohol.

Goal 2: Implement One Sleep Hygiene Strategy

Choose ONE from this list:

- Establish consistent bedtime and wake time (same time every day, even weekends)
- Make bedroom completely dark (blackout curtains or eye mask)
- Lower bedroom temperature to 65°F (18°C) or cooler
- Remove all screens from bedroom
- Create a 30-minute wind-down routine before bed

Why: Sleep affects everything. Starting here creates immediate benefits and supports all other changes.

Goal 3: Add One Stress-Reduction Practice

Choose ONE from this list:

- 5-10 minutes of deep breathing daily (morning or evening)
- 10-minute morning walk outside (bonus: gets morning light exposure)
- 5 minutes of journaling before bed

- Download a meditation app and do one guided session daily

Why: Stress worsens every symptom. Daily stress management is foundational.

Goal 4: Schedule Healthcare Appointments

If you do not have a healthcare provider you trust for menopause management:

- Research providers (gynecologists, menopause specialists, functional medicine doctors)
- Schedule an appointment (even if it is weeks away, get it on the calendar)

If you already have a provider:

- Schedule your appointment
- Prepare your list of symptoms and questions

Goal 5: Order Targeted Supplements or Products

Based on your top 3 symptoms, decide what you want to try:

- **For hot flashes:** NoPause Hot Flashes Support
- **For mood symptoms:** NoPause Mood Support
- **For sleep:** NoPause mood Support **or** Magnesium glycinate + L-theanine
- **For bone health:** Calcium + Vitamin D3 + K2
- **For brain fog:** Omega-3 fish oil + B-complex

Order these so you have them for Week 2.

Week 1 Success Markers:

- You tracked symptoms for 7 days
- You implemented one sleep hygiene improvement
- You practiced stress reduction daily
- You scheduled healthcare appointments if needed
- You ordered targeted supplements

Week 2: Add Nutrition and Supplements

Your Week 2 Goals

Continue tracking and build on Week 1 habits.

Goal 1: Continue Sleep and Stress Practices from Week 1

These should be becoming habits now. Stay consistent.

Goal 2: Make Three Nutrition Changes

Choose THREE from this list:

Blood Sugar Stability:

- Eat protein with every meal and snack
- Eliminate added sugar (desserts, sweetened beverages, candy)
- Replace refined grains with whole grains

Anti-Inflammatory Eating:

- Add 2 extra servings of vegetables daily
- Include fatty fish 2-3x this week
- Replace vegetable oil with avocado oil or olive oil

Reduce Triggers:

- Eliminate or reduce alcohol (aim for 3 or fewer drinks per week)
- Cut caffeine intake by half or eliminate after 12 PM
- Avoid spicy foods if they trigger hot flashes

Why: Nutrition directly impacts symptoms. These changes reduce inflammation, stabilize hormones, and eliminate common triggers.

Goal 3: Start Your Targeted Supplements

Begin the supplements you ordered:

138

- Follow label directions carefully
- Take consistently (set phone reminders if needed)
- Note any effects (positive or concerning) in your tracking

Remember: supplements take 4-12 weeks for full benefits. Be patient and consistent.

Goal 4: Add Movement

If you are not currently exercising regularly, start small:

- Take a 20-minute walk 3x this week
- Do 10 minutes of stretching or yoga daily
- Try 1 beginner strength training workout (bodyweight or light dumbbells)

If you already exercise regularly:

- Add 1 strength training session this week (or increase to 2 if you are doing 1)
- Ensure you are doing weight-bearing exercise

Goal 5: Review Your Tracking Data

At the end of Week 2, review your symptom tracking from Weeks 1-2:

- Are patterns emerging?
- Which lifestyle factors correlate with better or worse symptoms?
- How are the changes you made affecting how you feel?

Week 2 Success Markers:

- You continued sleep hygiene and stress practices
- You made 3 nutrition improvements
- You started targeted supplements consistently
- You added movement 3 times per week at least
- You reviewed your tracking and identified patterns

Week 3: Intensify Lifestyle Strategies

Your Week 3 Goals

You have built momentum. Now intensify your efforts.

Goal 1: Optimize Sleep Hygiene

Add 2-3 more sleep hygiene strategies:

- Implement a complete bedroom makeover (cool, dark, quiet)
- Perfect your bedtime routine (30-60 minutes of wind-down activities)
- Get morning light within 30 minutes of waking
- Eliminate screens 90 minutes before bed
- Take your NoPause Mood Support or magnesium glycinate supplements 30-60 minutes before bed

Goal 2: Expand Nutrition Improvements

Add 2-3 more nutrition strategies:

- Plan and prep meals for the week (meal prep Sunday)
- Increase vegetable intake to 5-7 servings daily
- Add fermented foods for gut health (yogurt, kefir, sauerkraut)
- Include flaxseeds or soy for phytoestrogens
- Hydrate adequately (half your body weight in ounces of water daily)

Goal 3: Increase Movement Frequency

- Strength training: 2 times this week (minimum)
- Cardiovascular activity: 3-5 times this week (walking, cycling, swimming)
- Daily movement: Take movement breaks every hour if you sit for work
- Add flexibility work: 10 minutes of stretching or yoga daily

Goal 4: Deepen Stress Management

Increase your stress-reduction practice:

- Extend meditation to 15-20 minutes daily
- Add breathwork: Practice 4-7-8 breathing 3x daily
- Schedule one activity purely for joy and relaxation this week
- Practice saying no to one commitment that drains you
- Connect with a friend or loved one

Goal 5: Environmental Toxin Reduction

Make 3 swaps:

- Replace plastic food storage with glass containers
- Switch to a cleaner personal care product (shampoo, deodorant, lotion)
- Filter your water (pitcher filter or install under-sink filter)
- Choose organic for your most frequently eaten produce
- Use natural cleaning products (vinegar, baking soda, castile soap)

Week 3 Success Markers:

- Sleep hygiene is fully optimized
- Nutrition is significantly improved
- You are exercising 5 days per week
- Stress management is a daily priority
- You made 3 environmental swaps

Week 4: Evaluate, Adjust, and Plan Next Steps

Your Week 4 Goals

This week is about evaluation and planning your long-term strategy.

Goal 1: Reassess Your Symptoms

Using the same rating scale from your baseline assessment, rate all symptoms again:

Compare your ratings:

- Which symptoms improved?
- Which symptoms are unchanged?
- Are any symptoms worse?
- How much have your top 3 priority symptoms improved (percentage)?

Realistic expectations after 4 weeks:

- Lifestyle changes: You should notice some improvements (better sleep, more energy, reduced hot flash frequency, improved mood)
- Supplements: Some benefits may be appearing, but full effects may take 8-12 weeks
- If you started hormones, you may see significant improvements already

Goal 2: Healthcare Provider Appointment

Have your appointment with your healthcare provider this week (or finalize plans if appointment is scheduled for next week).

Bring to your appointment:

- Your symptom tracking data (all 4 weeks)
- Your baseline and Week 4 symptom ratings
- List of supplements you are taking
- Your top 3 priority symptoms
- Questions about treatments you are considering

Discuss:

- Whether you are a candidate for bioidentical hormone therapy
- Whether you need any testing (thyroid, vitamin D, hormone levels, bone density)
- Whether your current treatment plan should be adjusted
- Any concerning symptoms
- Timeline for reevaluation

Goal 3: Decide on Hormones (If Applicable)

Based on your symptom severity, improvement so far, and conversation with your provider:

If symptoms improved 50% or more with lifestyle and supplements:

- Consider continuing current approach
- Monitor for another 4-8 weeks to see if improvements continue
- Hormones can always be added later if needed

If symptoms improved 20-40%:

- Consider adding hormones for additional relief
- Continue lifestyle and supplement strategies (they support hormone therapy)

If symptoms improved less than 20% or are still severely affecting quality of life:

- Strongly consider bioidentical hormone therapy
- This level of symptoms warrants more aggressive treatment
- Lifestyle and supplements alone may not be sufficient

Goal 4: Refine Your Plan

Based on what worked and what did not:

Keep doing:

- Any lifestyle change that helped
- Any supplement that seems beneficial
- Any practice that felt good or improved symptoms

Modify:

- Areas where you struggled (find easier alternatives)
- Strategies that did not seem to help (try different approaches)
- Timing or dosing of supplements if needed

Add:

- Additional treatments if symptoms remain problematic
- Hormones if you and your provider decided this is appropriate
- More advanced strategies for specific symptoms

Goal 5: Set Your Next 30-Day Goals

You have completed the Jumpstart Plan. Now set goals for the next 30 days:

Symptom goals:

- What additional improvement do you want to see?
- Which symptoms are you targeting next?

Lifestyle goals:

- What habits do you want to strengthen?
- What new practices do you want to add?

Treatment goals:

- Are you starting hormones?
- Are you trying additional supplements?
- Are you seeing specialists?

Week 4 Success Markers:

- You completed a full symptom reassessment
- You had your healthcare appointment (or have one scheduled)
- You made informed decisions about next steps
- You refined your plan based on results
- You set clear goals for the next 30 days

Tracking Tools and Templates

Daily Symptom Tracker

Create a simple daily log (paper journal, notes app, or spreadsheet):

Date: _____

Sleep:

- Time to bed: _____
- Time awake: _____
- Quality (1-10): _____
- Number of awakenings: _____

Hot Flashes:

- Daytime frequency: _____
- Nighttime frequency: _____
- Average severity (1-10): _____

Mood:

- Overall mood (1-10): _____
- Anxiety level (1-10): _____
- Energy level (1-10): _____

Cognitive:

- Brain fog (1-10): _____
- Memory (1-10): _____

Physical:

- Pain level (1-10): _____
- Overall well-being (1-10): _____

Lifestyle:

- Exercise: (type/duration)
- Stress management: (Y/N, what did you do?)
- Supplements taken: (Y/N)
- Alcohol: (servings)
- Caffeine: (servings, timing)

Notes:

- Anything unusual or noteworthy
- Foods that seemed to help or hurt
- Stressors or challenges
- Wins or positive observations

Weekly Progress Summary

At the end of each week, summarize:

Week ___:

Symptoms that improved:

_____

Symptoms that worsened or stayed the same: _____

Lifestyle wins: _____

Challenges faced: _____

Adjustments to make next week: _____

Overall feeling about this week (1-10): _____

What If Nothing Is Helping?

If you have completed this 30-day plan and seen minimal improvement, do not despair. This means you need additional support.

Next steps:

1. Rule out other conditions:

- Get comprehensive blood work (thyroid, vitamin D, vitamin B12, iron, complete metabolic panel)
- Ensure nothing else is contributing to symptoms

2. Try bioidentical hormones if you have not:

- Moderate to severe symptoms often require hormones for adequate relief
- Lifestyle and supplements support hormones but may not be sufficient alone

3. Add non-hormonal medications if hormones are not an option:

- SSRIs, SNRIs, gabapentin, or fezolinetant can provide significant relief

4. See a specialist:

- Menopause specialist
- Functional medicine practitioner
- Reproductive endocrinologist

5. Address underlying stress or trauma:

- Sometimes emotional work is necessary for physical healing
- Consider therapy, EMDR, or somatic therapies

6. Be patient:

- Some treatments take 3-6 months for full benefits
- Keep tracking and adjusting

Maintaining Your Progress Long-Term

The 30-Day Jumpstart creates momentum. Maintaining progress requires ongoing commitment, but it becomes easier as habits solidify.

Keys to long-term success:

1. Keep tracking intermittently: You do not need to track every day forever, but periodic tracking (one week per month) keeps you accountable and helps you notice if symptoms are creeping back.

2. Maintain lifestyle foundations: The habits you built—sleep hygiene, stress management, nutrition, exercise—are lifelong. They support you far beyond menopause.

3. Adjust treatments as needed: Your needs will change. Hormone doses may need adjustment. Supplement regimens may evolve. Stay in communication with your healthcare provider.

4. Do not abandon what works: If something helped, keep doing it. Many women stop treatments when they feel better, then symptoms return. Consistency matters.

5. Be kind to yourself: You will have weeks where you do not do everything perfectly. That is normal and okay. Progress, not perfection.

6. Celebrate your wins: Notice and acknowledge improvements. Celebrate feeling better. You deserve to thrive.

Your Journey Continues

This 30-Day Jumpstart Plan is just the beginning. You have the knowledge, tools, and strategies to manage your symptoms and optimize your well-being throughout perimenopause, menopause, and beyond.

The women who do best are those who:

- Stay informed and curious
- Advocate for themselves
- Are willing to experiment and adjust
- Maintain healthy lifestyle habits
- Seek support when needed
- Believe they deserve to feel good

You are one of those women. You picked up this handbook. You read this far. You are ready to take action.

Your transformation starts now.

ACTION STEPS

1. **Complete your baseline symptom assessment** before starting Week 1.
2. **Identify your top 3 priority symptoms** to focus your efforts.
3. **Follow the weekly plan systematically** (do not try to do everything at once).
4. **Track consistently** so you can measure progress objectively.
5. **Schedule your healthcare appointment** in Week 1 for Week 4.
6. **Order supplements or products** at the start so you have them when needed.
7. **Be patient with the process** (most interventions take 4-12 weeks for full benefit).
8. **Reassess at 30 days** and adjust your plan based on results.
9. **Commit to the journey** beyond 30 days—this is about lasting transformation.

"The 30-Day Jumpstart Plan gave me structure when I felt overwhelmed. I followed it step by step, tracked everything, and by Week 3, I noticed real improvements. At 30 days, my hot flashes were down 70%, I was sleeping better, and my mood was stable. Having a clear plan made all the difference."

— Renita, 47, Jamaica

CHAPTER 10

Walking Beside Her - A Guide for Partners

If you are reading this chapter, you care deeply about the woman in your life who is navigating perimenopause or menopause. You may have picked up this book because:

- She asked you to read it
- You want to understand what she is experiencing
- You feel confused or frustrated by changes in her mood, energy, or intimacy
- You want to help but do not know how
- Your relationship is struggling and you are looking for answers

Thank you for being here. Your support matters more than you may realize.

This chapter will help you understand what your partner is experiencing, how to support her effectively, and how to navigate this transition together as a team.

What You Need to Understand

This Is Real and Physical

The most important thing you need to know is this: **what your partner is experiencing is not "all in her head."**

Her symptoms are caused by dramatic hormonal shifts affecting her entire body, her brain, cardiovascular system, bones, muscles, metabolism, temperature regulation, sleep centers, and mood pathways.

When she says:

- "I cannot sleep", means her hormones are literally disrupting her sleep architecture
- "I feel anxious all the time", means declining progesterone has reduced her brain's calming neurotransmitters
- "I cannot think straight", means fluctuating estrogen is affecting her brain's metabolism and cognitive function
- "I have no energy", means multiple physiological changes are creating profound fatigue
- "I do not feel like myself", that is because her biochemistry has fundamentally changed

This is not weakness. This is not an excuse. This is biology.

The Symptoms Are Not About You

When she is irritable, withdrawn, or uninterested in intimacy, it is not because she is angry with you or no longer loves you (unless, of course, there are separate relationship issues).

Irritability: Hormonal fluctuations affect neurotransmitters that regulate mood and stress tolerance. She may snap at things that normally would not bother her.

Withdrawal: When she is exhausted from poor sleep, battling hot flashes, and struggling with anxiety or depression, she may have nothing left to give at the end of the day.

Low libido: Declining testosterone (yes, women need testosterone too) directly reduces sexual desire. Vaginal dryness and painful intercourse make intimacy physically uncomfortable. Fatigue and mood changes further diminish interest.

None of this reflects her feelings about you.

This Is Temporary But Can Last Years

Perimenopause typically lasts 4-8 years (sometimes longer). Once she reaches menopause (12 months without a period), some symptoms improve naturally as hormones stabilize, even though they remain low.

However, without treatment, some symptoms, particularly vaginal dryness, bone loss, and metabolic changes continue or worsen.

The good news: effective treatments exist. With the right support (medical and from you), most women can feel dramatically better.

Your role during these years is crucial.

She Needs Your Patience and Understanding

This transition is hard. She may not always handle it gracefully. She may be emotional, frustrated, short-tempered, or withdrawn.

What she needs most is for you to:

- Believe her when she says she is struggling
- Not take her symptoms personally
- Support her in seeking help
- Be patient during the process of finding solutions
- Remind her this is temporary and treatable

What she does not need:

- You to minimize her experience ("It is not that bad")
- You to offer unsolicited solutions ("Have you tried just relaxing?")
- You to compare her to other women ("My friend's wife did not have any problems")
- You to make her symptoms about you ("What about my needs?")
- You to pressure her about intimacy when she is not ready

How Perimenopause and Menopause May Be Affecting Her

Let me describe what she may be experiencing daily.

Sleep Disruption

Imagine waking up drenched in sweat 3-6 times per night, every night, for months or years. Your sheets are soaked. You are hot, then cold. You change your clothes. By the time you fall back asleep, you wake again.

This is not occasional poor sleep. This is chronic, severe sleep deprivation that affects everything, mood, cognition, energy, health, and relationships.

What you might notice: She is exhausted, forgetful, emotional, or irritable. She may nap during the day. She may fall asleep on the couch. She may drink excessive caffeine trying to function.

How you can help:

- Keep the bedroom cool (she needs it cooler than you probably want)
- Do not complain if she uses cooling sheets, fans, or opens windows even in winter
- Take over morning responsibilities if she had a terrible night
- Encourage her to prioritize sleep and seek treatment for night sweats
- Be patient with her fatigue

Hot Flashes

Picture this: You are sitting in a normal-temperature room when suddenly intense heat floods your body. Your face turns red. Sweat pours down your back and chest. Your heart races. You feel panicked and uncomfortable.

This happens 10-20 times per day (sometimes more). It happens during important meetings, social events, intimate moments, and in the middle of the night.

What you might notice: She suddenly strips off layers, fans herself, opens windows, or becomes flustered and uncomfortable. She may avoid social situations or feel embarrassed.

How you can help:

- Do not complain about the temperature (she is not doing this on purpose)
- Hand her a cold drink or damp cloth when she has a hot flash
- Do not draw attention to her flushing or sweating
- Support her in seeking treatment (hot flashes are very treatable)
- Be flexible if she needs to step outside or cool down during activities

Mood Changes and Anxiety

Hormonal fluctuations directly affect neurotransmitters, particularly serotonin (mood), GABA (calm), and dopamine (motivation and pleasure).

She may experience:
- Crying for no apparent reason
- Anxiety that was not there before
- Irritability and anger out of proportion to the situation
- Depression and hopelessness
- Mood swings,fine one moment, crying or angry the next

What you might notice: She seems like a different person emotionally. She may cry easily, snap at you, or seem withdrawn and sad.

How you can help:

- Recognize this is biochemical, not character failure
- Do not tell her to "calm down" or "stop being so emotional"
- Encourage her to seek help (therapy, hormones, medications, supplements)
- Be patient when she is emotional

- Tell her you love her and you are in this together
- Do not take her irritability personally (while also not accepting abuse—there is a line)

Brain Fog and Memory Problems

Estrogen is crucial for brain function. When it fluctuates or declines, many women experience:

- Forgetting words mid-sentence
- Walking into rooms and forgetting why
- Difficulty concentrating
- Trouble following conversations or complex information
- Forgetting appointments, tasks, or important information

This terrifies many women because they fear dementia. It is not dementia, it is temporary cognitive disruption from hormonal changes, and it typically improves with treatment.

What you might notice: She forgets things she normally would not. She seems distracted or confused. She may ask you the same question twice. She may struggle at work.

How you can help:

- Do not make jokes about her memory ("Getting old, huh?")
- Help with reminders for important tasks or appointments
- Be patient when she loses her train of thought
- Reassure her this is normal and treatable, not dementia
- Encourage her to seek treatment
- Pick up the slack when her cognitive function is struggling

Low Libido and Sexual Changes

This is often the most challenging aspect for partners to navigate.

Multiple factors affect her sexuality:

- **Declining testosterone** reduces desire
- **Vaginal dryness and atrophy** make intercourse painful

- **Fatigue** leaves no energy for intimacy
- **Mood changes** reduce interest in connection
- **Body image concerns** from weight gain or physical changes
- **Feeling "not like herself"** makes intimacy feel foreign

What you might notice: She rarely initiates intimacy. She declines your advances. She seems uninterested or avoidant. Intercourse may be uncomfortable for her.

How you can help (this is critical):

- **Do not pressure her or make her feel guilty**
- Recognize that low libido is a symptom, not a choice
- Support her in treating vaginal dryness (this is essential, painful sex kills desire)
- Expand your definition of intimacy beyond intercourse (touching, cuddling, kissing, massage)
- Talk openly about what feels good and what does not
- Be patient while she explores treatment options
- Focus on emotional connection, not just physical
- Consider couples counseling if this is significantly straining your relationship

Important: Pressuring her for sex when she is exhausted, in pain, or hormonally depleted will damage your relationship. Supporting her through this will strengthen it.

What She Needs From You

1. Believe Her

When she tells you she is struggling, believe her. Do not minimize, dismiss, or compare her to others.

Say this: "I believe you. This sounds really hard. What do you need from me?"

Not this: "You seem fine to me." "Other women do not complain this much." "Are you sure it is not just stress?"

2. Educate Yourself

You are reading this chapter, which is excellent. Keep going. Read the other chapters in this book. Learn about what she is experiencing. Understanding helps you have compassion.

3. Encourage Her to Seek Help

Many women try to "tough it out" because they have been told this is just aging or they do not want to complain.

Encourage her to:

- See a healthcare provider who specializes in menopause
- Try treatment (hormones, supplements, medications)
- Prioritize self-care (sleep, exercise, stress management)

Say this: "I want you to feel better. Let me help you find a doctor." "What can I do to support you in getting treatment?"

Not this: "Why do not you just go to the doctor?" (as if she is choosing to suffer)

4. Adjust Expectations

Your life together may need to shift during this transition:

- She may need more rest
- Social activities may need to be reduced
- Household responsibilities may need rebalancing
- Intimacy may need to be approached differently
- Patience will be required

This does not mean sacrificing your needs entirely, but it does mean being flexible and understanding.

5. Help Practically

Take tasks off her plate:

- Increase your share of household responsibilities
- Handle things that usually fall to her
- Let her rest when she needs to
- Take over bedtime routines with kids if applicable
- Run errands, cook meals, do laundry

Create a supportive environment:

- Keep the house cooler (accommodate her temperature needs)
- Be quiet in the morning if she had a terrible night
- Create time for her to exercise or practice stress management
- Encourage her to spend time with supportive friends

6. Be Patient With The Process

Finding the right treatment takes time. Hormones need adjustment. Supplements take weeks to work. Lifestyle changes require consistency.

There will be trial and error. What works for one woman may not work for her. Stay patient and encouraging throughout the process.

7. Communicate Openly

Do not let resentment build. Talk about how this transition is affecting both of you.

Use "I" statements: "I feel disconnected from you lately and I miss our closeness. How can we work on this together?"

Not blame: "You never want to be intimate anymore and it is ruining our relationship."

Ask her what she needs. Tell her what you need. Find compromises. Consider couples counseling if communication breaks down.

Navigating Intimacy During This Transition

Sexual changes are one of the most common relationship strains during menopause. Let us address this directly.

Why Her Libido Has Changed

It is not about you. Repeat this to yourself: **It is not about you.**

Her libido is affected by:

- Hormonal changes (low testosterone, low estrogen)
- Physical discomfort (vaginal dryness, pain during intercourse)
- Fatigue (she is exhausted from poor sleep)
- Mood changes (hard to feel desire when anxious or depressed)
- Body image issues (physical changes affect confidence)

These are physiological barriers, not emotional rejection.

What Not to Do

Do not:

- Pressure, guilt, or coerce her
- Make her feel broken or inadequate
- Complain about lack of sex in a way that makes her feel worse
- Compare her to how she used to be or other women
- Make everything about your needs
- Give up on physical connection entirely

What to Do Instead

1. Address the physical barriers first: Painful intercourse must be treated. Encourage her to:

- Use vaginal estrogen (remarkably safe and effective)
- Use high-quality lubricants
- See a pelvic health physical therapist if needed
- Try different positions that reduce discomfort

2. Redefine intimacy: Intimacy is not just intercourse. Expand your definition:

- Cuddling and holding each other
- Massage (giving and receiving)
- Kissing without expectation of sex
- Taking walks together
- Emotional connection and deep conversations
- Non-sexual physical touch throughout the day

3. Prioritize her pleasure: If intimacy does happen, focus on what feels good for her. This might mean more foreplay, different activities, or approaches that prioritize her arousal and comfort.

4. Be patient and encouraging: Libido often improves with treatment (particularly testosterone for women who are deficient). The process takes time.

5. Communicate without pressure: Talk about intimacy outside the bedroom. Ask her:

- What feels good and what does not?
- What would make intimacy more appealing?
- What barriers exist?
- How can you support her?

6. Consider professional help: Sex therapists or couples' counselors who specialize in sexual health can provide guidance for navigating this together.

Taking Care of Yourself

Supporting a partner through perimenopause or menopause can be emotionally draining. You have needs too.

It is okay to:

- Feel frustrated sometimes
- Wish things were different
- Miss aspects of your relationship

- Need support yourself

Take care of yourself:

- Talk to trusted friends (while respecting her privacy about details)
- Consider individual therapy if you are struggling
- Maintain your hobbies and interests
- Exercise and manage your stress
- Couples counseling can help both of you

Balance is key: Support her without sacrificing your own well-being entirely.

What Not to Say (And What to Say Instead)

Do not say: "You are overreacting." **Say instead:** "I can see you are really struggling. How can I help?"

Do not say: "Just relax, have a glass of wine, take a bubble bath." **Say instead:** "What would be most helpful for you right now?"

Do not say: "My friend's wife went through menopause and she was fine." **Say instead:** "Everyone's experience is different. What you are going through is real."

Do not say: "When are you going to be back to normal?" **Say instead:** "I am here for you through this transition, however long it takes."

Do not say: "What about my needs?" **Say instead:** "This is hard for both of us. Can we talk about how we both get our needs met?"

Do not say: "You have changed so much." **Say instead:** "I know this transition is hard. I love you and we will get through it together."

This Is a Partnership

Your partner is going through a profound biological transition. It is not easy for her, and it is not easy for you.

But here is the truth: How you show up during this time matters enormously.

Partners who are patient, understanding, supportive, and willing to learn often find their relationships deepen and strengthen through this transition.

Partners who are dismissive, selfish, or unsupportive often find their relationships suffer or end.

You have a choice about which partner you will be.

She will remember how you treated her during one of the hardest times of her life. Choose kindness. Choose patience. Choose partnership.

The good news: With proper treatment and support, she will feel better. This is not forever. But your response to her during this time may shape your relationship forever.

ACTION STEPS FOR PARTNERS

1. **Read this entire handbook** to truly understand what she is experiencing.
2. **Ask her what she needs** rather than assuming you know.
3. **Help her find a qualified healthcare provider** (research options, schedule appointments, go with her if she wants).
4. **Take tasks off her plate** to reduce her stress and create time for self-care.
5. **Be patient with her symptoms** and remember they are not about you.
6. **Keep the bedroom cool** and accommodate her temperature needs without complaint.
7. **Support treatment** (hormones, supplements, lifestyle changes) and give it time to work.
8. **Redefine intimacy** and do not pressure her sexually.
9. **Communicate openly and kindly** about how this transition is affecting both of you.
10. **Consider couples counseling** if the relationship is significantly strained.

11. **Take care of yourself too** so you can show up as a supportive partner.

"My husband read this chapter and it changed everything. He finally understood that my symptoms were not about him and that I was not choosing to be tired or irritable. He started helping more around the house, stopped complaining about the bedroom temperature, and supported me in getting treatment. Feeling like we were a team again made this transition so much more bearable."

Maria, 49, USA

PART IV

MOVING FORWARD WITH CONFIDENCE

CHAPTER 11

Moving Forward - Your Path to Thriving

You have reached the end of this handbook, but this is truly just the beginning of your journey to feeling better.

You now understand what is happening in your body. You know your treatment options, from lifestyle strategies to nutraceuticals to medications to bioidentical hormones. You have a 30-Day Jumpstart Plan. You know how to advocate for yourself and build your healthcare team.

Most importantly, you know that you do not have to suffer.

This final chapter provides two essential tools to support you moving forward: a practical 7-day Mediterranean meal plan to jumpstart your nutrition, and encouragement for the journey ahead.

The Mediterranean Diet for Hormone Health

Throughout this handbook, we have emphasized anti-inflammatory nutrition as foundational to managing perimenopausal and menopausal symptoms. The Mediterranean diet is one of the most researched, evidence-based eating patterns for reducing inflammation, supporting hormone balance, and promoting overall health.

The Mediterranean approach emphasizes:

- Abundant vegetables and fruits
- Whole grains
- Legumes and nuts
- Olive oil as the primary fat
- Fish and seafood regularly

- Moderate amounts of poultry and eggs
- Limited red meat
- Moderate wine (optional)
- Herbs and spices instead of salt

Research shows that Mediterranean-style eating reduces hot flashes, supports cardiovascular health, helps maintain healthy weight, reduces inflammation, supports brain health, and improves overall well-being during menopause.

Here is a practical 7-day meal plan to get you started.

7-Day Mediterranean Meal Plan

General Guidelines

Portions: These are general serving suggestions. Adjust based on your hunger, activity level, and individual needs. Focus on eating until satisfied, not stuffed.

Flexibility: Swap meals within the same category (any breakfast for another breakfast, any lunch for another lunch). Repeat favorites.

Preparation: Many components can be prepared in advance. Cook grains, roast vegetables, and prepare proteins ahead for easier assembly.

Hydration: Drink plenty of water throughout the day. Herbal tea is excellent. Limit caffeine to morning hours if it affects your sleep.

DAY 1

BREAKFAST: Greek Yogurt Bowl

- 1 cup plain Greek yogurt (protein and probiotics)
- 1/4 cup mixed berries (antioxidants)
- 2 tablespoons ground flaxseeds (lignans, omega-3s, fiber)
- 1 tablespoon chopped walnuts (healthy fats)
- Drizzle of honey (optional)
- Cinnamon to taste

LUNCH: Mediterranean Chickpea Salad

- 2 cups mixed greens (spinach, arugula, romaine)
- 3/4 cup chickpeas (protein and fiber)
- 1/2 cucumber, diced
- 1/2 cup cherry tomatoes, halved
- 1/4 cup red onion, thinly sliced
- 1/4 cup kalamata olives
- 2 tablespoons crumbled feta cheese
- Dressing: 2 tablespoons olive oil, 1 tablespoon lemon juice, oregano, salt, pepper

SNACK:

- 1/4 cup raw almonds
- 1 small apple

DINNER: Baked Salmon with Roasted Vegetables

- 4-5 oz wild-caught salmon, baked with lemon and dill
- 1 cup roasted broccoli and cauliflower (tossed in olive oil, garlic, lemon)
- 1/2 cup quinoa cooked in vegetable broth
- Side salad with olive oil and vinegar

DAY 2

BREAKFAST: Vegetable Omelet

- 2-3 eggs or egg whites
- Sautéed spinach, tomatoes, and mushrooms
- 1 oz feta cheese
- 1 slice whole grain toast with olive oil or avocado
- Fresh fruit on the side

LUNCH: Lentil and Vegetable Soup

- Hearty soup with lentils, carrots, celery, tomatoes, kale, garlic, herbs (make a big batch)
- 2 tablespoons ground flaxseeds stirred in

- Side of whole grain crackers or bread
- Small mixed greens salad with olive oil dressing

SNACK:

- Hummus (1/4 cup) with cucumber, carrots, and bell pepper slices

DINNER: Grilled Chicken with Mediterranean Vegetables

- 4-5 oz grilled chicken breast with herbs and lemon
- Roasted eggplant, zucchini, and red peppers drizzled with olive oil and balsamic vinegar
- 1/2 cup whole grain couscous or bulgur wheat
- Fresh tomato and cucumber salad

DAY 3

BREAKFAST: Overnight Oats

- 1/2 cup rolled oats soaked overnight in unsweetened almond milk
- 1 tablespoon chia seeds
- 1 tablespoon ground flaxseeds
- 1/4 cup berries
- 1 tablespoon almond butter
- Cinnamon and vanilla extract

LUNCH: Tuna and White Bean Salad

- 1 can wild-caught tuna (in water or olive oil)
- 3/4 cup white beans (cannellini)
- Mixed greens
- Cherry tomatoes
- Red onion
- Fresh parsley
- Dressing: Olive oil, lemon juice, Dijon mustard

SNACK:

- 1/4 cup walnuts
- 1 orange

DINNER: Shrimp and Vegetable Stir-Fry

- 4-6 oz shrimp sautéed in olive oil with garlic
- Abundant vegetables: broccoli, snap peas, bell peppers, carrots
- Serve over 1/2 cup brown rice or quinoa
- Season with herbs, lemon, red pepper flakes

DAY 4

BREAKFAST: Mediterranean Scramble

- 2-3 eggs scrambled with olive oil
- Sautéed spinach, tomatoes, and onions
- 2 tablespoons crumbled feta
- Whole grain toast
- Sliced avocado

LUNCH: Mediterranean Grain Bowl

- 1/2 cup quinoa or farro
- 3/4 cup chickpeas roasted with cumin and paprika
- Roasted vegetables (zucchini, red peppers, red onion)
- Handful of arugula
- Tahini dressing (tahini, lemon juice, garlic, water to thin)
- Sprinkle of pumpkin seeds

SNACK:

- Greek yogurt with a handful of berries and 1 tablespoon ground flaxseeds

DINNER: Baked White Fish with Vegetables

- 5-6 oz white fish (cod, halibut, or sea bass) baked with tomatoes, olives, capers, garlic, olive oil

- Steamed green beans with lemon and almonds
- Small baked sweet potato with olive oil and herbs
- Side salad

DAY 5

BREAKFAST: Smoothie Bowl

- Blend: 1 cup unsweetened almond milk, 1 cup spinach, 1/2 banana, 1/2 cup frozen berries, 1 scoop protein powder (optional), 1 tablespoon almond butter, 1 tablespoon ground flaxseeds
- Top with: sliced fruit, chia seeds, coconut flakes, nuts

LUNCH: Greek Salad with Grilled Chicken

- Large Greek salad: romaine, cucumbers, tomatoes, red onion, bell peppers, kalamata olives, feta cheese
- 4 oz grilled chicken breast
- Dressing: Olive oil, red wine vinegar, oregano, garlic
- Whole grain pita on the side

SNACK:

- Celery sticks with 2 tablespoons almond butter
- Small handful of grapes

DINNER: Turkey Meatballs with Marinara and Vegetables

- Turkey meatballs made with ground turkey, egg, whole grain breadcrumbs, garlic, herbs
- Marinara sauce (tomato-based, no added sugar)
- Serve over spiralized zucchini noodles or whole grain pasta (small portion)
- Side of roasted Brussels sprouts with olive oil

DAY 6

BREAKFAST: Avocado Toast with Eggs

- 1-2 slices whole grain or sourdough bread, toasted
- 1/2 avocado mashed with lemon, salt, red pepper flakes
- 2 poached or soft-boiled eggs on top
- Side of cherry tomatoes
- Fresh fruit

LUNCH: Mediterranean Lentil Salad

- 1 cup cooked green or brown lentils
- Diced cucumbers, tomatoes, red onion, bell peppers
- Fresh parsley and mint
- Crumbled feta cheese
- Dressing: Olive oil, lemon juice, garlic
- Serve over mixed greens

SNACK:

- Apple slices with 2 tablespoons tahini or almond butter

DINNER: Grilled Salmon with Herb Sauce

- 5 oz grilled or baked salmon
- Fresh herb sauce (parsley, cilantro, olive oil, lemon, garlic)
- Roasted asparagus and cherry tomatoes
- 1/2 cup wild rice or quinoa
- Arugula salad with lemon and olive oil

DAY 7

BREAKFAST: Shakshuka (Eggs in Tomato Sauce)

- Tomato-based sauce with bell peppers, onions, garlic, cumin, paprika
- 2 eggs poached directly in the sauce
- Fresh herbs (parsley or cilantro)
- Whole grain bread for dipping

- Side of sliced cucumber

LUNCH: Sardine and Avocado Toast

- 2 slices whole grain bread, toasted
- 1/2 avocado mashed
- 1 can sardines (in olive oil or water)
- Squeeze of lemon, red pepper flakes
- Large side salad with olive oil and vinegar dressing

SNACK:

- 1/4 cup mixed nuts (almonds, walnuts, pistachios)
- 1 pear

DINNER: Mediterranean Stuffed Peppers

- Bell peppers stuffed with mixture of ground turkey or chicken, quinoa, diced tomatoes, spinach, herbs, a little feta
- Baked until tender
- Side of roasted zucchini and eggplant
- Small green salad

Meal Plan Tips and Modifications

Make It Work for You

Vegetarian: Replace fish and poultry with additional legumes, tofu, tempeh, or eggs. Increase nuts and seeds for protein.

Vegan: Eliminate dairy and eggs. Use plant-based yogurt, nutritional yeast instead of cheese, tofu scrambles instead of eggs.

Gluten-free: Choose gluten-free whole grains (quinoa, rice, buckwheat, millet) and gluten-free bread options.

Time-saving: Prepare components in advance. Cook grains and legumes in bulk. Pre-chop vegetables. Use quality canned or frozen items (canned beans, frozen vegetables, frozen fish).

Key Principles

Protein at every meal: Stabilizes blood sugar and reduces cravings. Aim for 20-30 grams per meal.

Abundant vegetables: Target 5-7 servings daily. Include at both lunch and dinner, add to breakfast when possible.

Healthy fats: Olive oil, nuts, seeds, avocado, fatty fish. These are anti-inflammatory and hormone-supportive.

Whole grains in moderation: 1/2 cup cooked grains per meal is appropriate for most women. Adjust based on your activity level and how your body responds.

Limit added sugar: Use fruit for sweetness. Occasional honey or maple syrup in small amounts is fine.

Stay hydrated: Water, herbal teas, and sparkling water are your friends.

Foods to Emphasize

Daily:

- Vegetables (especially leafy greens and cruciferous vegetables)
- Olive oil
- Nuts and seeds
- Whole grains
- Legumes
- Fresh herbs and spices

3-4 times per week:

- Fatty fish (salmon, sardines, mackerel)
- Eggs
- Greek yogurt or another fermented dairy

Occasionally:

- Poultry
- Red meat (small portions, grass-fed when possible)
- Natural sweets (dark chocolate, fruit-based desserts)

Beyond the Meal Plan: Your Journey Forward

This Is Not the End—It Is the Beginning

You have the knowledge. You have the tools. You have the meal plan. Now comes the implementation and the commitment to yourself.

Remember these truths:

1. You deserve to feel good. Perimenopause and menopause symptoms are treatable. You do not have to accept suffering as inevitable.

2. Small, consistent actions create transformation. You do not need to be perfect. You just need to be consistent with the basics: nutrition, movement, sleep, stress management, and appropriate treatments.

3. Progress is not linear. You will have good weeks and hard weeks. That is normal. What matters is that you keep moving forward.

4. You are not alone. Millions of women worldwide are experiencing exactly what you are experiencing. Reach out for support from healthcare providers, friends, family, support groups, or online communities.

5. This transition is temporary. The journey to transition from perimenopause to menopause can last years, however, with proper support and treatment, you can feel dramatically better, often within weeks to months. Your symptoms will become manageable and you will thrive through this season.

6. You are still you. Hormonal changes do not define you. The woman that you are, strong, capable, worthy has now been empowered to navigate this biological transition, with knowledge and resilience.

Your Next Steps

This week:

- Implement the 7-day meal plan (or start with 3-4 days)
- Continue or begin the 30-Day Jumpstart Plan from Chapter 9
- Schedule healthcare appointments if you have not already
- Order NoPause products or other quality supplements for your priority symptoms
- Share the "Walking Beside Her" chapter with your partner if applicable

This month:

- Complete your baseline symptom tracking
- Make lifestyle changes systematically (not all at once)
- Start targeted treatments
- Track your progress

This year:

- Optimize all six lifestyle pillars (nutrition, movement, sleep, stress, gut health, toxin reduction)
- Find the right treatment combination for your unique needs
- Adjust and refine as you learn what works for your body
- Support other women navigating this transition
- Celebrate your progress

When You Need Extra Support

Resources:

- North American Menopause Society (menopause.org): Reliable information and provider directory
- International Menopause Society (imsociety.org): Global resources and information
- NoPause website: (NoPausemd.com) For physician-formulated supplements (Hot Flashes Support and Mood Support)

- Online menopause communities: Connect with other women (while being discerning about advice)

If symptoms are severe or not improving:

- Seek care from a menopause specialist
- Consider comprehensive hormone testing
- Explore functional or integrative medicine approaches
- Do not hesitate to try different providers until you find one who helps
- Remember that finding the right treatment combination can take time

A Final Word of Encouragement

Navigating this transitional period in your life can be distressing. My own personal struggles unfolded in an unusual place. While performing a surgical procedure, I nearly fainted in the operating room, when I was overwhelmed by the heat from a severe hot flash. I experienced the unrelenting hot flashes, the night sweats, and the exhaustion. I understand the frustration of feeling like your body has betrayed you and the fear that you will never feel like yourself again.

But I also know the other side. I know what it feels like to wake up refreshed after a full night of sleep. To go an entire day without a hot flash. To feel mentally sharp and emotionally stable. To have energy and vitality. To feel like myself again. Frankly I do not have time to pause, my assignment to humanity, demands that I am fully present and in the best mental and physical health, to function optimally.

That is possible for you too.

The journey may take time. You may need to try different approaches. You will likely need to combine lifestyle strategies with targeted treatments. But relief is available, and you deserve to have it.

You are not being dramatic. You are not weak. You are not asking for too much.

You are navigating a profound biological transition, and you are seeking the support you need to feel good during and after that transition. That is wisdom, not weakness.

Move forward with confidence. You have the knowledge. You have the tools. You have the plan.

Now take the first step. And then the next. And then the next.

Your transformation awaits.

FINAL ACTION STEPS

1. **Keep this handbook** as your reference guide and return to it when you need guidance or encouragement.
2. **Start the 7-day Mediterranean meal plan** this week.
3. **Begin the 30-Day Jumpstart Plan** (or continue if you already started).
4. **Order NoPause Hot Flashes Support or Mood Support** (or other quality supplements) for your priority symptoms.
5. **Schedule your healthcare appointments** and be prepared with your symptoms list and questions.
6. **Share relevant chapters** with your partner, family, or friends who could benefit.
7. **Join a support community** (online or in-person) for encouragement and connection.
8. **Track your progress** so you can see improvements objectively.
9. **Celebrate every victory**: improved sleep, fewer hot flashes, better mood, more energy.
10. **Remember: You deserve to thrive, not just survive, through this transition.**

"One year ago, I was suffering daily with hot flashes, insomnia, anxiety, and brain fog. I felt like I was losing myself. Today, after implementing the strategies in this handbook, Mediterranean-style eating, strength training, stress management, NoPause Hot Flashes Support and Mood Support, and bioidentical hormones, I feel better

than I have in years. If you are reading this and struggling, please know: relief is possible. Do not give up on yourself. You deserve to feel good."

Angella, 43, USA

THE NoPAUSE SOLUTION

You do not have to pause your life during perimenopause and menopause.

You can feel vibrant, energetic, mentally sharp, emotionally stable, and physically strong.

You can sleep through the night. You can think clearly. You can feel like yourself.

You can thrive.

That is the NoPause Solution.

Welcome to your transformation.

GLOSSARY

The NoPause Solution Handbook

A

Adaptogen
A natural substance that helps the body adapt to stress and promotes balance in bodily systems. Examples include ashwagandha and rhodiola.

Amenorrhea
The absence of menstrual periods. Primary amenorrhea is when menstruation has never occurred; secondary amenorrhea is when periods stop after having been regular.

Androgen
A group of hormones, including testosterone and DHEA, that play a role in male traits and reproductive activity. Women also produce androgens in smaller amounts.

Anovulation
A menstrual cycle in which the ovary does not release an egg. This becomes more common during perimenopause.

Antioxidant
A substance that protects cells from damage caused by free radicals. Examples include vitamins C and E.

Ashwagandha (Withania somnifera)
An adaptogenic herb used in traditional medicine to reduce stress, anxiety, and menopausal symptoms.

B

Bioidentical Hormones
Hormones that are chemically identical to those produced naturally by the human body. Often derived from plant sources and used in hormone replacement therapy.

BHRT (Bioidentical Hormone Replacement Therapy)
Treatment using bioidentical forms of estrogen, progesterone, and sometimes testosterone to relieve menopausal symptoms.

Biochanin A
An isoflavone found in red clover that has phytoestrogenic properties and may help reduce hot flashes.

Black Cohosh (Actaea racemosa)
A plant native to North America, traditionally used to treat menopausal symptoms, particularly hot flashes and mood changes.

Bone Density
The amount of bone mineral in bone tissue. Bone density decreases after menopause due to declining estrogen levels, increasing the risk of osteoporosis.

Brain Fog
A term describing cognitive difficulties including memory problems, difficulty concentrating, and mental cloudiness. Common during perimenopause and menopause.

C

Cardiovascular Disease
Diseases affecting the heart and blood vessels. Risk increases after menopause due to declining estrogen levels.

Climacteric
The period of life when fertility and sexual activity are in decline. In women, this includes perimenopause, menopause, and postmenopause.

Compounded BHRT
Custom-formulated bioidentical hormone therapy prepared by a compounding pharmacy according to a healthcare provider's prescription.

Corpus Luteum
A temporary structure in the ovary that forms after ovulation and produces progesterone. Its function declines during perimenopause.

Cortisol
A hormone produced by the adrenal glands in response to stress. Chronic elevation can worsen menopausal symptoms.

D

DHEA (Dehydroepiandrosterone)
A hormone produced by the adrenal glands that serves as a precursor to estrogen and testosterone. Levels decline with age.

Dyspareunia
Painful sexual intercourse, often caused by vaginal dryness and atrophy during menopause.

E

Early Menopause
Menopause occurring between ages 40 and 45. This is earlier than the average age of 51-52 years.

Endocrine System
The system of glands that produce and secrete hormones to regulate body functions.

Endometrium
The lining of the uterus that thickens each month and is shed during menstruation. After menopause, the endometrium becomes thin.

Estradiol (E2)
The most potent form of estrogen produced primarily by the ovaries during reproductive years. Levels decline significantly during menopause.

Estriol (E3)
A weak form of estrogen that increases during pregnancy. Sometimes used in bioidentical hormone therapy.

Estrogen
A group of hormones primarily responsible for female sexual characteristics and reproductive function. The three main types are estradiol, estrone, and estriol.

Estrogen Dominance
A condition where estrogen levels are high relative to progesterone levels. Common during perimenopause when ovulation becomes irregular.

Estrone (E1)
A weak form of estrogen that becomes the predominant estrogen after menopause. Produced mainly by fat tissue.

F

Fennel (Foeniculum vulgare)
An herb with phytoestrogenic properties used to help manage menopausal symptoms.

Fenugreek (Trigonella foenum-graecum)
An herb traditionally used to support hormonal balance and libido.

Follicle
A small sac in the ovary containing an immature egg. The number and quality of follicles decline with age.

Follicle-Stimulating Hormone (FSH)
A hormone produced by the pituitary gland that stimulates the ovaries to produce eggs and estrogen. FSH levels rise during perimenopause and menopause as the ovaries become less responsive.

Formononetin
An isoflavone found in red clover with phytoestrogenic properties.

G

Genitourinary Syndrome of Menopause (GSM)
A collection of symptoms related to decreased estrogen affecting the vagina, vulva, and lower urinary tract. Symptoms include vaginal dryness, burning, irritation, and urinary problems. Formerly called vaginal atrophy.

Genistein
An isoflavone found in soy and red clover with phytoestrogenic effects.

H

Hormone
A chemical messenger produced by glands that travels through the bloodstream to regulate various body functions.

Hormone Replacement Therapy (HRT)
Treatment using hormones (estrogen with or without progesterone) to relieve menopausal symptoms and reduce health risks associated with estrogen decline.

Hot Flash (Hot Flush)
A sudden feeling of intense heat, often accompanied by sweating and flushing of the face and upper body. The most common symptom of menopause.

HPA Axis (Hypothalamic-Pituitary-Adrenal Axis)
The interaction between the hypothalamus, pituitary gland, and adrenal glands that regulates stress response and many body processes.

Hypothalamus
A region of the brain that controls body temperature, hunger, thirst, and hormone production. Plays a role in hot flashes.

I

Isoflavones
Plant compounds with weak estrogenic properties found in soy, red clover, and other legumes. Used to help manage menopausal symptoms.

Irregular Periods
Menstrual cycles that vary in length, flow, or frequency. Very common during perimenopause.

L

Lemon Balm (Melissa officinalis)
An herb in the mint family used to reduce anxiety, improve mood, and promote sleep.

Libido
Sexual desire. Often decreases during menopause due to hormonal changes, vaginal dryness, and other factors.

L-Theanine
An amino acid found in tea that promotes relaxation, reduces stress and anxiety, and improves sleep quality without causing drowsiness.

Luteinizing Hormone (LH)
A hormone produced by the pituitary gland that triggers ovulation and stimulates the ovaries to produce estrogen and progesterone.

M

Magnesium Glycinate
A highly absorbable form of magnesium that supports mood, reduces anxiety, improves sleep, and helps maintain bone health.

Mediterranean Diet
An eating pattern emphasizing fruits, vegetables, whole grains, legumes, nuts, olive oil, and fish. Associated with reduced menopausal symptoms and improved health outcomes.

Melatonin
A hormone that regulates sleep-wake cycles. Production can be affected during menopause.

Menopause
The point when menstrual periods have stopped for 12 consecutive months, marking the end of reproductive years. Average age is 51-52 years.

Menopause Rating Scale (MRS)
A standardized questionnaire used to assess the severity of menopausal symptoms.

Menstrual Cycle
The monthly hormonal cycle in which the uterus prepares for pregnancy. Cycles become irregular during perimenopause.

Metabolic Syndrome
A cluster of conditions (increased blood pressure, high blood sugar, excess abdominal fat, abnormal cholesterol) that increase risk of heart disease and diabetes. More common after menopause.

Milk Thistle (Silybum marianum)
An herb known for liver support and antioxidant properties, sometimes used to support hormonal balance.

N

Night Sweats
Episodes of excessive sweating during sleep, often requiring clothing or bedding changes. A form of hot flash that occurs at night.

Nutraceutical
A product derived from food sources that provides health benefits beyond basic nutrition. Includes dietary supplements, herbal products, and functional foods.

O

Osteopenia
Lower than normal bone density but not as severe as osteoporosis. Increases risk of developing osteoporosis.

Osteoporosis
A condition in which bones become weak and brittle due to loss of bone density, increasing fracture risk. Risk increases significantly after menopause due to estrogen decline.

Ovarian Reserve
The number and quality of eggs remaining in the ovaries. Declines with age.

Ovary
The female reproductive organ that produces eggs and hormones (primarily estrogen and progesterone).

Ovulation
The release of an egg from the ovary, typically occurring mid-cycle. Becomes irregular and eventually stops during perimenopause.

P

Perimenopause
The transition period before menopause when hormone levels fluctuate and symptoms begin. Can last 4-10 years, with an average of 4-6 years.

Phytoestrogen
Plant-derived compounds that have weak estrogenic effects in the body. Found in soy, red clover, flaxseeds, and other plants.

Pituitary Gland
A small gland at the base of the brain that produces hormones regulating other glands, including FSH and LH.

Post-menopause
The years following menopause, lasting for the rest of a woman's life.

Premature Ovarian Insufficiency (POI)
Also called premature menopause, this occurs when the ovaries stop functioning normally before age 40.

Progesterone
A hormone produced by the ovaries after ovulation that prepares the uterus for pregnancy and balances estrogen's effects.

Progestin
A synthetic form of progesterone used in some hormone replacement therapies and birth control.

Provera (Medroxyprogesterone Acetate)
A synthetic progestin used in some hormone replacement therapies. Not bioidentical to natural progesterone.

R

Red Clover (Trifolium pratense)
A plant rich in isoflavones used to help reduce hot flashes and other menopausal symptoms.

S

Sage (Salvia officinalis)
An herb with phytoestrogenic properties traditionally used to reduce hot flashes, night sweats, and excessive perspiration during menopause.

Selective Serotonin Reuptake Inhibitor (SSRI)
A class of antidepressant medications that can also help reduce hot flashes and improve mood during menopause.

Serotonin
A neurotransmitter that regulates mood, sleep, and body temperature. Levels can be affected by hormonal changes during menopause.

Sleep Disturbance
Difficulty falling asleep, staying asleep, or poor sleep quality. Very common during perimenopause and menopause.

Surgical Menopause
Menopause that occurs when both ovaries are surgically removed (bilateral oophorectomy), causing an immediate cessation of hormone production.

T

Testosterone
An androgen hormone that plays a role in libido, energy, muscle mass, and bone density. Women produce small amounts, primarily from the ovaries and adrenal glands. Levels decline with age.

Thyroid
A gland in the neck that produces hormones regulating metabolism. Thyroid disorders become more common around menopause and can mimic menopausal symptoms.

Transdermal
Administered through the skin, such as hormone patches, gels, or creams. This route bypasses the liver and may have different effects than oral hormones.

U

Urinary Incontinence
Loss of bladder control, ranging from occasional leakage to complete inability to control urination. Can worsen after menopause due to tissue changes.

Uterus
The hollow muscular organ where a fetus develops during pregnancy. The lining (endometrium) is shed monthly during menstruation.

V

Vaginal Atrophy
Now called Genitourinary Syndrome of Menopause (GSM). Thinning, drying, and inflammation of the vaginal walls due to decreased estrogen.

Vaginal Dryness
Lack of adequate moisture in the vagina, causing discomfort, itching, and painful intercourse. Common after menopause due to declining estrogen.

Vasomotor Symptoms (VMS)
Hot flashes and night sweats caused by changes in the body's temperature regulation system.

W

Weight Gain
An increase in body weight, particularly around the abdomen, commonly occurring during perimenopause and menopause due to hormonal changes, decreased metabolism, and muscle loss.

Withania somnifera
The scientific name for ashwagandha, an adaptogenic herb used to manage stress, anxiety, and menopausal symptoms.

X

Xenoestrogens
Synthetic or natural chemical compounds that mimic estrogen in the body. Found in plastics, pesticides, and personal care products. May disrupt normal hormonal balance.

Note: This glossary provides definitions for terms used throughout The NoPause Solution Handbook. Terms are defined in simple, accessible language to help readers understand medical and scientific concepts related to perimenopause and menopause.

CITATIONS FOR THE NoPAUSE SOLUTION HANDBOOK

A Physician's Integrative Guide Through Perimenopause and Menopause

Note: Citations are organized by chapter and formatted in AMA (American Medical Association) style.

PART I: UNDERSTANDING WHAT'S HAPPENING

CHAPTER 1: Perimenopause vs. Menopause - What's the Difference?

1. Harlow SD, Gass M, Hall JE, et al. Executive summary of the Stages of Reproductive Aging Workshop +10: addressing the unfinished agenda of staging reproductive aging. *Menopause.* 2012;19(4):387-395.
2. Santoro N, Roeca C, Peters BA, Neal-Perry G. The menopause transition: signs, symptoms, and management options. *J Clin Endocrinol Metab.* 2021;106(1):1-15.
3. Gold EB, Colvin A, Avis N, et al. Longitudinal analysis of the association between vasomotor symptoms and race/ethnicity across the menopausal transition: Study of Women's Health Across the Nation. *Am J Public Health.* 2006;96(7):1226-1235.

CHAPTER 2: Understanding Your Hormones

1. Davis SR, Wahlin-Jacobsen S. Testosterone in women—the clinical significance. *Lancet Diabetes Endocrinol.* 2015;3(12):980-992.
2. Prior JC. Progesterone for treatment of symptomatic menopausal women. *Climacteric.* 2018;21(4):358-365.
3. Santoro N, Randolph JF Jr. Reproductive hormones, and the menopause transition. *Obstet Gynecol Clin North Am.* 2011;38(3):455-466.
4. Burger HG, Hale GE, Robertson DM, Dennerstein L. A review of hormonal changes during the menopausal transition: focus

on findings from the Melbourne Women's Midlife Health Project. *Hum Reprod Update*. 2007;13(6):559-565.

CHAPTER 3: Why This Happens - The Science Behind the Symptoms

1. Freeman EW, Sammel MD, Lin H, Nelson DB. Associations of hormones and menopausal status with depressed mood in women with no history of depression. *Arch Gen Psychiatry*. 2006;63(4):375-382.
2. Maki PM, Thurston RC. Menopause and brain health: hormonal changes are only part of the story. *Front Neurol*. 2020; 11:562275.
3. Thurston RC, Joffe H. Vasomotor symptoms and menopause: findings from the Study of Women's Health across the Nation. *Obstet Gynecol Clin North Am*. 2011;38(3):489-501.
4. Weber MT, Maki PM, McDermott MP. Cognition and mood in perimenopause: a systematic review and meta-analysis. *J Steroid Biochem Mol Biol*. 2014; 142:90-98.

PART II: TREATMENT OPTIONS

CHAPTER 4: HRT and BHRT - The Complete Guide

1. Manson JE, Chlebowski RT, Stefanick ML, et al. Menopausal hormone therapy, and health outcomes during the intervention and extended poststopping phases of the Women's Health Initiative randomized trials. *JAMA*. 2013;310(13):1353-1368.
2. Rossouw JE, Anderson GL, Prentice RL, et al. Risks and benefits of estrogen plus progestin in healthy postmenopausal women: principal results from the Women's Health Initiative randomized controlled trial. *JAMA*. 2002;288(3):321-333.
3. Anderson GL, Limacher M, Assaf AR, et al. Effects of conjugated equine estrogen in postmenopausal women with hysterectomy: the Women's Health Initiative randomized controlled trial. *JAMA*. 2004;291(14):1701-1712.
4. The NAMS 2017 Hormone Therapy Position Statement Advisory Panel. The 2017 hormone therapy position statement of The North American Menopause Society. *Menopause*. 2017;24(7):728-753.

5. Pinkerton JV, Aguirre FS, Blake J, et al. The 2017 hormone therapy position statement of The North American Menopause Society. *Menopause*. 2017;24(7):728-753.
6. Hodis HN, Mack WJ, Henderson VW, et al. Vascular effects of early versus late postmenopausal treatment with estradiol. *N Engl J Med*. 2016;374(13):1221-1231.
7. Files JA, Ko MG, Pruthi S. Bioidentical hormone therapy. *Mayo Clin Proc*. 2011;86(7):673-680.
8. American College of Obstetricians and Gynecologists. ACOG Practice Bulletin No. 141: management of menopausal symptoms. *Obstet Gynecol*. 2014;123(1):202-216.
9. Cirigliano M. Bioidentical hormone therapy: a review of the evidence. *J Women's Health (Larchmt)*. 2007;16(5):600-631.
10. L'Hermite M. Bioidentical hormone therapy: practical recommendations. *Gynecol Endocrinol*. 2013;29 Suppl 1:41-47.
11. Schmidt PJ, Ben Dor R, Martinez PE, et al. Effects of estradiol withdrawal on mood in women with past perimenopausal depression: a randomized clinical trial. *JAMA Psychiatry*. 2015;72(7):714-726.
12. Santen RJ, Allred DC, Ardoin SP, et al. Postmenopausal hormone therapy: an Endocrine Society scientific statement. *J Clin Endocrinol Metab*. 2010;95(7 Suppl 1): s1-s66.

CHAPTER 5: Nutraceuticals - The NoPause Solution

NoPause Hot Flashes Support Ingredients:

SAGE (Salvia officinalis)

1. Bommer S, Klein P, Suter A. First time proof of sage's tolerability and efficacy in menopausal women with hot flushes. *Adv Ther*. 2011;28(6):490-500.
2. Moradi M, Rafieian-Kopaei M, Karami M. The Effect of Salvia Officinalis on Hot Flashes in Postmenopausal Women: A Systematic Review and Meta-Analysis. *Przegl Menopauzalny*. 2023;22(2):71-78.
3. Dadfar F, Bamdad K. The effect of Salvia officinalis extract on symptoms of flushing, night sweats, sleep disorders, and

score of forgetfulness in postmenopausal women. *Int J Reprod Biomed.* 2019;17(4):267-274.

RED CLOVER (Trifolium pratense)

4. Kanadys W, Barańska A, Błaszczuk A, et al. Evaluation of Clinical Meaningfulness of Red Clover (Trifolium pratense L.) Extract to Relieve Hot Flushes and Menopausal Symptoms in Peri- and Post-Menopausal Women: A Systematic Review and Meta-Analysis of Randomized Controlled Trials. *Nutrients.* 2021;13(4):1258.
5. Myers SP, Vigar V. Effects of a standardised extract of Trifolium pratense (Promensil) at a dosage of 80mg in the treatment of menopausal hot flushes: a systematic review and meta-analysis. *Phytomedicine.* 2017; 24:141-147.
6. Hidalgo LA, Chedraui PA, Morocho N, Ross S, San Miguel G. The effect of red clover isoflavones on menopausal symptoms, lipids, and vaginal cytology in menopausal women: a randomized, double-blind, placebo-controlled study. *Gynecol Endocrinol.* 2005;21(5):257-264.
7. Lambert MNT, Thorup AC, Hansen ESS, Jeppesen PB. Combined Red Clover isoflavones and probiotics potently reduce menopausal vasomotor symptoms. *PLoS One.* 2017;12(6): e0176590.

FENNEL SEED (Foeniculum vulgare)

8. Rahimikian F, Rahimi R, Golzareh P, Bekhradi R, Mehran A. Effect of Foeniculum vulgare Mill. (fennel) on menopausal symptoms in postmenopausal women: a randomized, triple-blind, placebo-controlled trial. *Menopause.* 2017;24(9):1017-1021.
9. Yaralizadeh M, Abedi P, Najar S, Namjoyan F, Saki A. Effect of Foeniculum vulgare (fennel) vaginal cream on vaginal atrophy in postmenopausal women: A double-blind randomized placebo-controlled trial. *Maturitas.* 2016; 84:75-80.

ASHWAGANDHA (Withania somnifera)

10. Gopal S, Ajgaonkar A, Kanchi P, et al. Effect of an ashwagandha (Withania Somnifera) root extract on climacteric symptoms in women during perimenopause: A randomized, double-blind, placebo-controlled study. *J Obstet Gynaecol Res*. 2021;47(12):4414-4425.
11. Chandrasekhar K, Kapoor J, Anishetty S. A prospective, randomized double-blind, placebo-controlled study of safety and efficacy of a high-concentration full-spectrum extract of ashwagandha root in reducing stress and anxiety in adults. *Indian J Psychol Med*. 2012;34(3):255-262.
12. Salve J, Pate S, Debnath K, Langade D. Adaptogenic and anxiolytic effects of ashwagandha root extract in healthy adults: a double-blind, randomized, placebo-controlled clinical study. *Cureus*. 2019;11(12): e6466.

FOLATE, VITAMIN E, VITAMIN D3

13. Kennedy DO. B vitamins and the brain: mechanisms, dose and efficacy—a review. *Nutrients*. 2016;8(2):68.
14. Palacios C, Kostiuk LK, Peña-Rosas JP. Vitamin D supplementation for women during pregnancy. *Cochrane Database Syst Rev*. 2019;7(7):CD008873.
15. Rizvi S, Raza ST, Ahmed F, Ahmad A, Abbas S, Mahdi F. The role of vitamin E in human health and some diseases. *Sultan Qaboos Univ Med J*. 2014;14(2):e157-e165.

NoPause Mood Support Ingredients:

L-THEANINE

16. Hidese S, Ogawa S, Ota M, et al. Effects of L-Theanine Administration on Stress-Related Symptoms and Cognitive Functions in Healthy Adults: A Randomized Controlled Trial. *Nutrients*. 2019;11(10):2362.
17. Williams JL, Everett JM, D'Cunha NM, et al. The Effects of Green Tea Amino Acid L-Theanine Consumption on the Ability to Manage Stress and Anxiety Levels: a Systematic Review. *Plant Foods Hum Nutr*. 2020;75(1):12-23.

18. Sarris J, Byrne GJ, Cribb L, et al. L-theanine in the adjunctive treatment of generalized anxiety disorder: A double-blind, randomised, placebo-controlled trial. *J Psychiatr Res*. 2019;110:31-37.
19. Rao TP, Ozeki M, Juneja LR. In Search of a Safe Natural Sleep Aid. *J Am Coll Nutr*. 2015;34(5):436-447.

ASHWAGANDHA (see citations 10-12 above)

MILK THISTLE (Silybum marianum)

20. Dietz BM, Hajirahimkhan A, Dunlap TL, Bolton JL. Botanicals and their bioactive phytochemicals for women's health. *Pharmacol Rev*. 2016;68(4):1026-1073.
21. Greenlee H, Abascal K, Yarnell E, Ladas E. Clinical applications of Silybum marianum in oncology. *Integr Cancer Ther*. 2007;6(2):158-165.

LEMON BALM (Melissa officinalis)

22. Cases J, Ibarra A, Feuillère N, Roller M, Sukkar SG. Pilot trial of Melissa officinalis L. leaf extract in the treatment of volunteers suffering from mild-to-moderate anxiety disorders and sleep disturbances. *Med J Nutrition Metab*. 2011;4(3):211-218.
23. Haybar H, Javid AZ, Haghighizadeh MH, Valizadeh E, Mohaghegh SM, Mohammadzadeh A. The effects of Melissa officinalis supplementation on depression, anxiety, stress, and sleep disorder in patients with chronic stable angina. *Clin Nutr ESPEN*. 2018; 26:47-52.

FENUGREEK (Trigonella foenum-graecum)

24. Steels E, Rao A, Vitetta L. Physiological aspects of male libido enhanced by standardized Trigonella foenum-graecum extract and mineral formulation. *Phytother Res*. 2011;25(9):1294-1300.
25. Rao A, Steels E, Inder WJ, Abraham S, Vitetta L. Testofen, a specialised Trigonella foenum-graecum seed extract reduces age-related symptoms of androgen decrease, increases

testosterone levels, and improves sexual function in healthy aging males in a double-blind randomised clinical study. *Aging Male*. 2016;19(2):134-142.

MAGNESIUM GLYCINATE

26. Boyle NB, Lawton C, Dye L. The effects of magnesium supplementation on subjective anxiety and stress—a systematic review. *Nutrients*. 2017;9(5):429.
27. Arab A, Rafie N, Amani R, Shirani F. The role of magnesium in sleep health: a systematic review of available literature. *Biol Trace Elem Res*. 2023;201(1):121-128.
28. Tarleton EK, Littenberg B, MacLean CD, Kennedy AG, Daley C. Role of magnesium supplementation in the treatment of depression: a randomized clinical trial. *PLoS One*. 2017;12(6):e0180067.

B VITAMINS (B3, B6, B12)

29. Kennedy DO. B vitamins and the brain: mechanisms, dose and efficacy—a review. *Nutrients*. 2016;8(2):68.
30. Mikkelsen K, Stojanovska L, Apostolopoulos V. The Effects of Vitamin B in Patients with Depression. *Curr Med Chem*. 2016;23(38):4317-4337.
31. Balk EM, Raman G, Tatsioni A, Chung M, Lau J, Rosenberg IH. Vitamin B6, B12, and folic acid supplementation and cognitive function: a systematic review of randomized trials. *Arch Intern Med*. 2007;167(1):21-30.

VITAMIN D3 (see citation 14 above)

32. Anglin RE, Samaan Z, Walter SD, McDonald SD. Vitamin D deficiency and depression in adults: systematic review and meta-analysis. *Br J Psychiatry*. 2013; 202:100-107.

ADDITIONAL GENERAL NUTRACEUTICAL REFERENCES

33. Franco OH, Chowdhury R, Troup J, et al. Use of plant-based therapies and menopausal symptoms: a systematic review and meta-analysis. *JAMA*. 2016;315(23):2554-2563.

34. Sánchez-Borrego R, Mendoza N, Beltrán E, et al. Complementary methods for menopause symptom management: a systematic review. *Women's Midlife Health*. 2020; 6:7.

CHAPTER 6: Other Effective Treatments

1. Geller SE, Studee L. Botanical, and dietary supplements for menopausal symptoms: what works, what does not. *J Women's Health (Larchmt)*. 2005;14(7):634-649.
2. Duijts SF, van Beurden M, Oldenburg HS, et al. Efficacy of cognitive behavioral therapy and physical exercise in alleviating treatment-induced menopausal symptoms in patients with breast cancer: results of a randomized, controlled, multicenter trial. *J Clin Oncol*. 2012;30(33):4124-4133.
3. Nonhormonal management of menopause-associated vasomotor symptoms: 2015 position statement of The North American Menopause Society. *Menopause*. 2015;22(11):1155-1174.
4. Loprinzi CL, Sloan J, Stearns V, et al. Newer antidepressants and gabapentin for hot flashes: an individual patient pooled analysis. *J Clin Oncol*. 2009;27(17):2831-2837.
5. Guttuso T Jr, Kurlan R, McDermott MP, Kieburtz K. Gabapentin's effects on hot flashes in postmenopausal women: a randomized controlled trial. *Obstet Gynecol*. 2003;101(2):337-345.
6. Simon JA, Portman DJ, Kaunitz AM, et al. Low-dose paroxetine 7.5 mg for menopausal vasomotor symptoms: two randomized controlled trials. *Menopause*. 2013;20(10):1027-1035.

CHAPTER 7: Lifestyle as Medicine

1. Daley A, Stokes-Lampard H, Thomas A, MacArthur C. Exercise for vasomotor menopausal symptoms. *Cochrane Database Syst Rev*. 2014;(11):CD006108.
2. Reed SD, Guthrie KA, Newton KM, et al. Menopausal quality of life: RCT of yoga, exercise, and omega-3 supplements. *Am J Obstet Gynecol*. 2014;210(3):244.e1-244.e11.

3. Elavsky S, McAuley E. Physical activity and mental health outcomes during menopause: a randomized controlled trial. *Ann Behav Med*. 2007;33(2):132-142.
4. North American Menopause Society. The role of local vaginal estrogen for treatment of vaginal atrophy in postmenopausal women: 2007 position statement of The North American Menopause Society. *Menopause*. 2007;14(3 Pt 1):355-369.
5. Avis NE, Coeytaux RR, Levine B, Isom S, Morgan T. Trajectories of response to acupuncture for menopausal vasomotor symptoms: the Acupuncture in Menopause Study. *Menopause*. 2017;24(2):171-179.
6. Berin E, Hammar M, Lindblom H, Lindh-Åstrand L, Spetz Holm AC. Resistance training for hot flushes in postmenopausal women: a randomised controlled trial. *Maturitas*. 2019;126:55-60.

PART III: YOUR ACTION PLAN

CHAPTER 8: Nutrition for Hormone Health

1. Trichopoulou A, Costacou T, Bamia C, Trichopoulos D. Adherence to a Mediterranean diet and survival in a Greek population. *N Engl J Med*. 2003;348(26):2599-2608.
2. Estruch R, Ros E, Salas-Salvadó J, et al. Primary prevention of cardiovascular disease with a Mediterranean diet supplemented with extra-virgin olive oil or nuts. *N Engl J Med*. 2018;378(25):e34.
3. Samieri C, Sun Q, Townsend MK, et al. The association between dietary patterns at midlife and health in aging: an observational study. *Ann Intern Med*. 2013;159(9):584-591.
4. Veronese N, Stubbs B, Noale M, et al. Adherence to a Mediterranean diet is associated with lower incidence of frailty: a longitudinal cohort study. *Clin Nutr*. 2018;37(5):1492-1497.
5. Asghari G, Mirmiran P, Yuzbashian E, Azizi F. A systematic review of diet quality indices in relation to obesity. *Br J Nutr*. 2017;117(8):1055-1065.
6. Carr MC. The emergence of the metabolic syndrome with menopause. *J Clin Endocrinol Metab*. 2003;88(6):2404-2411.

7. Messina M. Soy and health update: evaluation of the clinical and epidemiologic literature. *Nutrients*. 2016;8(12):754.
8. Bauer J, Biolo G, Cederholm T, et al. Evidence-based recommendations for optimal dietary protein intake in older people: a position paper from the PROT-AGE Study Group. *J Am Med Dir Assoc*. 2013;14(8):542-559.

CHAPTER 9: Exercise and Movement

1. Daley A, Macarthur C, Stokes-Lampard H, McManus R, Wilson S, Mutrie N. Exercise participation, body mass index, and health-related quality of life in women of menopausal age. *Br J Gen Pract*. 2007;57(535):130-135.
2. Simkin-Silverman LR, Wing RR, Boraz MA, Kuller LH. Lifestyle intervention can prevent weight gain during menopause: results from a 5-year randomized clinical trial. *Ann Behav Med*. 2003;26(3):212-220.
3. Kohrt WM, Bloomfield SA, Little KD, Nelson ME, Yingling VR; American College of Sports Medicine. American College of Sports Medicine Position Stand: physical activity and bone health. *Med Sci Sports Exerc*. 2004;36(11):1985-1996.
4. Asikainen TM, Kukkonen-Harjula K, Miilunpalo S. Exercise for health for early postmenopausal women: a systematic review of randomised controlled trials. *Sports Med*. 2004;34(11):753-778.
5. Nelson ME, Rejeski WJ, Blair SN, et al. Physical activity and public health in older adults: recommendation from the American College of Sports Medicine and the American Heart Association. *Circulation*. 2007;116(9):1094-1105.

CHAPTER 10: Walking Beside Her - A Guide for Partners

1. Trompeter SE, Bettencourt R, Barrett-Connor E. Sexual activity and satisfaction in healthy community-dwelling older women. *Am J Med*. 2012;125(1):37-43.e1.
2. Kingsberg SA, Wysocki S, Magnus L, Krychman ML. Vulvar and vaginal atrophy in postmenopausal women: findings from the REVIVE (REal Women's VIews of Treatment Options for Menopausal Vaginal ChangEs) survey. *J Sex Med*. 2013;10(7):1790-1799.

3. Parish SJ, Hahn SR. Hypoactive sexual desire disorder: a review of epidemiology, biopsychology, diagnosis, and treatment. *Sex Med Rev.* 2016;4(2):103-120.

PART IV: MOVING FORWARD

CHAPTER 11: Moving Forward - Your Path to Thriving (Including Mediterranean Meal Plan)

1. Willett WC, Sacks F, Trichopoulou A, et al. Mediterranean diet pyramid: a cultural model for healthy eating. *Am J Clin Nutr.* 1995;61(6 Suppl):1402S-1406S.
2. Bach-Faig A, Berry EM, Lairon D, et al. Mediterranean diet pyramid today. Science and cultural updates. *Public Health Nutr.* 2011;14(12A):2274-2284.
3. Grosso G, Buscemi S, Galvano F, et al. Mediterranean diet and cancer: epidemiological evidence and mechanism of selected aspects. *BMC Surg.* 2013;13 Suppl 2:S14.
4. Martinez-Gonzalez MA, Bes-Rastrollo M. Dietary patterns, Mediterranean diet, and cardiovascular disease. *Curr Opin Lipidol.* 2014;25(1):20-26.

ADDITIONAL GENERAL REFERENCES

For general menopause information used throughout multiple chapters:

1. North American Menopause Society. Menopause Practice: A Clinician's Guide. 6th ed. North American Menopause Society; 2019.
2. Shifren JL, Gass ML; NAMS Recommendations for Clinical Care of Midlife Women Working Group. The North American Menopause Society recommendations for clinical care of midlife women. *Menopause.* 2014;21(10):1038-1062.
3. Stuenkel CA, Davis SR, Gompel A, et al. Treatment of symptoms of the menopause: an Endocrine Society clinical practice guideline. *J Clin Endocrinol Metab.* 2015;100(11):3975-4011.

NOTE ON CITATIONS

All clinical claims, statistics, and treatment recommendations in this handbook are supported by the peer-reviewed medical literature cited above. Where personal clinical experience and observations are shared, they are identified as such in the text.

For readers interested in exploring these topics further, the complete citations are provided here in AMA (American Medical Association) format, which is standard for medical publications.

ABOUT THE AUTHOR

Dr. Ivanah Thomas is a medical doctor, philanthropist, entrepreneur, author, and motivational speaker. She holds four doctoral degrees in fields as varied as medicine, clinical psychology, philosophy, and theology. She also holds a master's degree in business administration. Her long and distinguished career in the health care industry spans well over three decades, starting out as a registered nurse.

Her speaking acumen has taken her to the United Nations several times to speak on issues impacting girls and women, globally.

Fueled by her devotion to the improvement of humanity, she has developed a perimenopause line of products, called NoPause Health Solutions, to assist women naturally through their perimenopause and menopause journey.

She's a committed God's girl and remains focused on improving the health and wellbeing of humanity.

CONNECT WITH THE AUTHOR

I would love to hear from you. Please connect with me.

Website
www.nopausehealthsolutions.com

Facebook
www.facebook.com/profile.php?id=61583610900289

Instagram
www.instagram.com/nopauseofficial

TikTok
www.tiktok.com/@nopauseofficial

Substack
www.substack.com/@nopausehealthsolutions

LinkedIn
www.linkedin.com/in/ivanah-thomas-41303b351

Email
nopausemd@gmail.com